MEDICINES MANAGEMENT
FOR NURSING ASSOCIATES

2nd Edition

MEDICINES MANAGEMENT
FOR NURSING ASSOCIATES

Christina Roulston

Miriam Davies

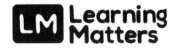

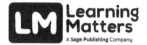

Learning Matters
A Sage Publishing Company
1 Oliver's Yard
55 City Road
London EC1Y 1SP

Sage Publications Inc.
2455 Teller Road
Thousand Oaks, California 91320

Sage Publications India Pvt Ltd
B 1/I 1 Mohan Cooperative Industrial Area
Mathura Road
New Delhi 110 044

Sage Publications Asia-Pacific Pte Ltd
3 Church Street
#10-04 Samsung Hub
Singapore 049483

Library of Congress Control Number: 2023947921

British Library Cataloguing in Publication Data

A catalogue record for this book is available from the British Library

Editor: Martha Cunneen
Development editor: Sarah Turpie
Senior project editor: Chris Marke
Marketing manager: Ruslana Khatagova
Project management: TNQ Tech Pvt. Ltd.
Cover design: Wendy Scott
Typeset by: TNQ Tech Pvt. Ltd.

ISBN 978-1-5296-2300-0
ISBN 978-1-5296-2301-7 (pbk)

Contents

About the authors   ix
Acknowledgements   x

Introduction   1

1   Legal and professional considerations for medicines management   5

2   The human body, ageing and the disease process   25

3   Principles of pharmacology   43

4   Safe medicines administration   59

5   Numeracy skills for drug calculations   81

6   Medication management in the modern age   119

7   Case studies: Applying principles to practice   137

Glossary   171
References   179
Index   185

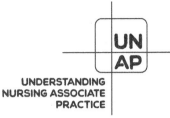

UN AP

UNDERSTANDING
NURSING ASSOCIATE
PRACTICE

Supporting you through your nursing associate training & career

UNDERSTANDING NURSING ASSOCIATE PRACTICE is a series uniquely designed for trainee nursing associates.

Each book in the series is:
- Mapped to the NMC standards of proficiency for nursing associates
- Affordable
- Full of practical activities & case studies
- Focused on clearly explaining theory & its application to practice

Other books in the series include:

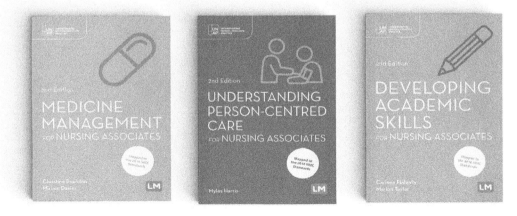

Visit
uk.sagepub.com/UNAP
to see the full collection

About the authors

Christina Roulston, RGN, Cert Ed ODP, BSc (Hons), PG Cert Sexual health, PG Cert Education, MA (Ed)

Tina has been a Lecturer at the University of Chester within the Faculty of Health, Medicine and Society since 2017. Prior to this, Tina had 20 years of adult nursing roles within the fields of day surgery and urology in secondary care as well as practice nurse roles in primary care. This experience was gained in both NHS, private and military care environments. Tina is the Programme Lead for Nursing associate students at the University of Chester, ensuring teaching provision supports learners' development. Tina primarily teaches the evidence-based underpinning practice, including medicine management for trainees.

Miriam Davies, BN (Hons), PG Dip SCPHN, PG Dip Professional Education, MSc

Miriam is a Lecturer at the University of Salford within the School of Health and Society. She has an adult nursing background within the fields of surgery and oncology. She later specialised in public health, working as a health visitor and continues to practise in this field. Her particular areas of clinical interest include child development, health promotion, medicines management and evidence-based practice.

Miriam primarily teaches pre-registration nursing, alongside involvement in postgraduate programmes, such as specialist community public health and masters in nursing. She has been actively involved with university research projects as well as curriculum design and planning for both nursing associate and pre-registration nursing programmes.

Acknowledgements

The authors would like to thank Eleanor Rivers for her enthusiastic and comprehensive support for the duration of the first edition's development. We would like to thank the editor, Laura Walmsley, for her support and guidance on the book's pedagogical features in line with the Understanding Nursing Associate Practice series.

We would like to thank our reviewer, Deborah Robertson, for her timely and detailed feedback and suggestions. We acknowledge that any errors or inaccuracies within this text are our own.

We are particularly grateful to the Resuscitation Council (UK) in acknowledgement of copyright permission for their anaphylactic treatment algorithm. In addition, the 'Malnutrition Universal Screening Tool' ('MUST') is reproduced with the kind permission of the British Association for Parenteral and Enteral Nutrition (BAPEN), 2011.

Finally, the authors would like to thank our University of Chester colleagues, families and friends for their 'you can do it' attitude and support in seeing this text through to completion; in particular, Katie Mansfield-Loynes for her initial 'nudge' to develop teaching resources into this text.

Introduction

What is medicines management?

Medicines management *encompasses the entire way that medicines are selected, procured, delivered, prescribed, administered and reviewed to optimise the contribution that medicines make to producing informed and desired outcomes of patient care* (Audit Commission, 2001).

Why is medicines management important?

There is a requirement for those working in healthcare to understand how to use medicines safely, economically, ethically and within the law, and to demonstrate compliance with national and local policies and employer guidelines. Paramount is the need to be aware and work within Employer's scope of practice for the Nursing associate role, adhering to their policies and procedures as these may well vary from organisation to organisation. Increasingly, the term 'medicines optimisation' (RPS, 2013) is being used to underline the requirement for person-centred care to obtain the maximum benefit for individual patients with the minimum of risk. This philosophy encourages patients to be partners in the choice of medicines and therapies, and in doing so improves patient compliance and adherence to treatments.

Who is this book for?

The nursing associate is a highly trained support role delivering effective, safe and responsive nursing care. The role requires you to work independently, within defined parameters, to deliver care in line with an agreed plan. As such, you will need to have a breadth of knowledge and skills to serve local health populations in a range of settings.

This book, as part of a Learning Matters series, is intended as a guide for nursing associates to equip you with the essential knowledge and skills required to safely administer medications in practice. It is mapped against the Nursing and Midwifery Council (NMC), *Standards of proficiency for nursing associates* (NMC, 2018a).

About the book

This book has been designed to be used for self-directed study to explore the core knowledge required to safely manage and administer medicines across the fields of nursing and the age continuum. It will allow consideration of the current discourse within modern pharmacology and demystify the nursing associate's role in medicines management as part of the wider healthcare team.

Pharmaceutical knowledge of regularly encountered medicines and the requirements for safe administration are an area of practice that causes trainee nursing associates a great deal of anxiety. It is an area of practice that you may well have had varying degrees of participation and responsibility. This book is designed as a systematic text that will explore medicines management with specific nursing associate accountability and is an accessible size to refer to within practice.

Book structure

The book is divided into seven easy-to-read chapters. The content and learning objectives of each chapter reflect the foundation degree study requirements for trainee nursing associates.

Chapter 1 discusses legal and professional issues underpinning medicines management to ensure ethical and accountable medicines administration. It explores the key legislation governing the supply, storage, dispensing, administering and disposing of drugs. It discusses accountability, responsibility and vicarious liability, and explores the principles of risk in medicines management. In addition, the standards of proficiency for medicines management for nursing associates are explained.

Chapter 2 is an introduction to the integrated anatomy and physiology of body systems necessary to ensure homoeostasis, with consideration of the effects of disease and ageing on the human body. In addition, basic pathophysiology is provided to allow understanding of the signs and symptoms that affect the service user, along with an explanation of infection control mechanisms.

Chapter 3 helps you understand the pharmacological aspects of medicines. This chapter discusses the pharmacokinetics of medicines, including the absorption, distribution, metabolism and excretion of drugs, along with factors that affect these, and the routes of administration. The pharmacodynamics are discussed, explaining the biotransformation of drugs for you to both understand these concepts and be able to explain to service users and their care givers.

Chapter 4 describes the role of the nursing associate in the safe administration of medicines, including accurate patient checks, the 'rights' of administration and the importance of communication and documentation in this context. It discusses mental capacity and competence in consent, patient concordance issues, adverse reactions, anaphylaxis and escalation requirements.

Chapter 5 provides an overview of the mathematical principles required to accurately and safely perform drug dose calculations. It provides the methods required to complete unit conversions and calculate drug dosages to allow for safe administration across the lifespan and fields of nursing.

Chapter 6 explores medicines management in the modern age, with regard to future opportunities and threats to healthcare, and its impact on medicines optimisation. It discusses the approval process for new drugs, an introduction to complementary therapies to assist with symptom control, including pain management. It highlights the misuse of medications, including antibiotic resistance and the opioid crisis, as well as vaccine hesitancy.

Chapter 7 explores field-specific care environments, allowing the application of theory to practice with a range of case studies to allow you to practise drug dose calculations and examine medicines management implications.

Requirements for the NMC standards of proficiency for nursing associates

The Nursing and Midwifery Council (NMC, 2018a) has established standards of proficiency to be met by applicants to different parts of the register, and these are the standards it considers necessary for safe and effective practice. This book is structured so that it will help you to understand and meet the proficiencies required for entry to the NMC register as a nursing associate. The relevant proficiencies are presented at the start of each chapter so that you can clearly see which ones the chapter addresses. The proficiencies have been designed to be generic, so they apply to all fields of nursing and all care settings. This is because all nursing associates must be able to meet the needs of any person they encounter in their practice, regardless of their stage of life or health challenges, whether these are mental, physical, cognitive or behavioural.

This book includes the latest standards for 2018 onwards, taken from the *Standards of proficiency for nursing associates* (NMC, 2018a).

Apprenticeship standard for nursing associate - ST0827

This standard (Institute for Apprenticeships and Technical Education, 2022) sets out the occupational duties, with the skills, knowledge and behaviours outlined, that individuals would need to demonstrate to obtain an accredited award approved by the NMC to allow registration. It specifies within it the requirements for safe and effective administration and optimisation of medicines in accordance with local and national policies. More details can be found at the Institute for Apprenticeships and Technical Education: *Nursing Associate (NMC) (ST0827)*; https://www.instituteforaprrenticeships.org/apprenticeship-standards/nursing-associate-nmc-2018-v1-1

Learning features

Textbooks can be intimidating and learning from reading text is not always easy. However, this series has been designed specifically to help the nursing associate learn from the books within it. By using a number of learning features throughout the books, they will help you develop your understanding and ability to apply theory to practice, while remaining engaging and breaking the text up into manageable chunks. This book contains activities, case studies, theory summary boxes, further reading, useful websites and other materials to enable you to participate in your own learning. The book cannot provide all the answers, but instead provides a good outline of the important information and helps you to build a framework for your own learning.

Throughout the book you will discover activities and case studies designed to assist you to link the theory presented with your practice. You may wish to include completed activities and reflections as part of your continuing professional development portfolio. In each chapter, you will discover words or terms highlighted in bold print where they first occur. Definitions of these can be found in the Glossary at the end of the book. In addition, at the end of each chapter will be highlighted resources, or sources of further reading to assist you to deepen your knowledge and understanding of the issues being discussed.

We hope you enjoy this book and find it a useful tool to aid you to develop your skill and confidence in medicines management.

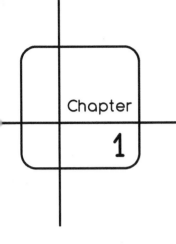

Chapter 1

Legal and professional considerations for medicines management

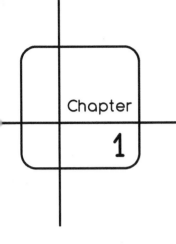

NMC STANDARDS OF PROFICIENCY FOR NURSING ASSOCIATES

This chapter will address the following platforms and proficiencies:

Platform 1 Being an accountable professional

1.1   understand and act in accordance with the Code (NMC, 2018b): Professional standards of practice and behaviour for nurses, midwives and nursing associates, and fulfil all registration requirements.

1.2   understand and apply relevant legal, regulatory and governance requirements, policies and ethical frameworks, including any mandatory reporting duties, to all areas of practice.

1.3   understand the importance of courage and transparency and apply the duty of candour (NMC, 2022), recognising and reporting any situations, behaviours or errors that could result in poor care outcomes.

Platform 4 Working in teams

4.1   demonstrate an awareness of the roles, responsibilities and scope of practice of different members of the nursing and interdisciplinary team, and their own role within it.

Platform 5 Improving safety and quality of care

5.1   understand and apply the principles of health and safety legislation and regulations and maintain safe work and care environments.

5.6   understand and act in line with local and national organisational frameworks, legislation and regulations to report risks, and implement actions as instructed, following up and escalating as required.

5.7   understand what constitutes a near miss, a serious adverse event, a critical incident and a major incident.

Chapter aims

After reading this chapter, you will be able to:

- understand the legal, regulatory and governance requirements for medicines management;
- understand the ethical frameworks of healthcare professionals in medicines management.

Introduction

Case study: Mary

You are a trainee nursing associate on a practice learning opportunity in the Accident and Emergency Department where Mary is attending, having fallen and broken her arm. As part of a holistic assessment, Mary has declared that she does not take any regular medications and is not allergic to anything. The department is busy, with several small children making a fuss and noise from an open window. Mary confides that she is glad she cannot have another baby at present, what with being on the pill. She later discloses that she has been suffering with anxiety for the last few months and has had occasional panic attacks. She has started smoking cannabis to relieve symptoms as this seems to help. She asks you to close the window otherwise she will have to use her inhaler which she takes when her hay fever is bad. You are concerned that there has been a misunderstanding in communication between the healthcare team and Mary regarding medication usage.

Mary's case study is a perfect example of the importance of medicines management and raises several issues you may encounter in your practice. Throughout this chapter, we will refer to Mary's case study and address the concerns identified within it.

This chapter sets out the relevant legal, regulatory and professional duties in all areas of practice for you as a nursing associate. Responsibilities include following governing policies, ethical frameworks and reporting procedures. Nursing associates must adhere to the *Code of conduct* as outlined by the Nursing and Midwifery Council (NMC, 2018b), specific standards for administration of medication (HEE, 2017; RPS, 2023), as well as local policies and employer expectations. In addition, as with all citizens, nursing associates are governed by the legislation surrounding medicines. This chapter will explore the legal and professional rationale for appropriate medicines management. It is important to remember that trainee nursing associates are not allowed to give any medicine to a service user unless assisting a registered nurse and must be actively supervised when involved with anything to do with medicines management. This is unless administration is agreed as part of an healthcare assistant role and is supported by Organisational medicine policy and indemnity. Once you become registered, you will need to abide by the ethical, professional, regulatory and employer requirements of your role. This chapter will help you to understand and feel confident in doing this by first defining what a medicine is and outlining your responsibilities and accountability. Next, the chapter describes the various pieces of legislation that regulate all aspects of medicines management, and finally it explores the roles of the multidisciplinary team within medicines management.

What is a medicine?

As you discovered when reading Mary's case study at the beginning of this chapter, we commonly use and hear a variety of terms when discussing healthcare with our service users and we may hold different perspectives on what constitutes a medicine. Therefore, let us start with an activity to help you reflect on your current knowledge of what a medical product is and identify the terms you have used and heard other professionals use when describing them.

Activity 1.1   Critical thinking

- What does the term 'medicine' mean?
- What should you take into consideration when coming up with your definition?

Complete this activity to develop your critical thinking abilities.

An outline answer is given at the end of this chapter.

If you take a moment to define what the term 'medicine' means, you may find that this is more difficult than it appears at first. Many of us may immediately think of the humble paracetamol tablet taken to relieve a headache or the antihistamine taken to relieve hay fever as examples; we may be more uncertain about including the vitamin tablet obtained from a health-food shop, the contraceptive implant, a wound dressing impregnated with a healing solution, a nicotine patch bought to alleviate cravings while giving up smoking or the herbal concoction obtained from complementary therapists.

We may additionally discover that we are using the terms 'medicine', 'drugs', 'tablets' and 'pills' interchangeably without considering their meaning or the connotations associated with them. In practice, in environments we may be familiar with when doing a 'medicine' round with the drug trolley, we ask our patients what tablets they regularly take and whether they are allergic to any medications. This common healthcare language does not take into consideration any negative connotations or service users' perceptions. As a society, we tend to use the terms 'drug abuse', 'drug dealer' or 'drug smuggler' when describing the illegal or more seedy aspects of medication use, this can relate to both prescribed and illicit medications. As a nursing associate, one of your roles will be to ensure concordance, which will be discussed in a later chapter, and as such you need to inspire confidence in treatment regimes. Your patients need to have confidence that their medication will have the desired therapeutic benefit and, as such, your terminology is important. In addition, when considering the meaning of the term 'medicine', it is important to consider the patient's perspective. Are substances being taken recreationally, regularly or as symptoms dictate, or as a health food or cosmetic? As with all healthcare, minimising misinterpretations and communicating effectively are key to ensuring high standards of care and are essential to ensure safe and appropriate medications management.

Historically, people have used products derived from a variety of sources to alter bodily functions. Ancient cultures utilised substances from animal, plant and mineral sources for the purpose of relieving symptoms. In the early part of the twentieth century, a manufacturer could introduce a medicine on to the market with very few restrictions. In the United Kingdom, the law was fundamentally changed following the use of thalidomide during pregnancy, a drug marketed as a sleeping tablet but used widely as a relief for morning sickness, which had tragic consequences with an increase in the number of babies born with major limb deformities. In modern times, the control of the discovery, production and utilisation of these substances has required scrutiny, definition and regulation.

The Human Medicines Regulations 2012 define a medicinal product as

> *any substance or combination of substances presented as having properties of preventing or treating disease in human beings; or any substance or combination of substances that may be used by or administered to human beings with a view to: restoring, correcting or modifying a physiological function by exerting a pharmacological, immunological or metabolic action, or making a medical diagnosis.*

Furthermore, the European Council Directive 2004/27/EC states that a substance is a medicinal product if it is distributed as having properties for treating or preventing disease. This recognises that a product may also be defined as a something else, such as a cosmetic or health food. The European Parlimentary Research Service (2015) state 'Food products or food supplements, medical devices, biocides and cosmetics are called borderline products'.

Law and the nursing associate

You have chosen a career as a nursing associate to meet the needs of individuals with various health and social care needs, not because you wish to study law. However, in the current climate of increased litigation, a legal awareness that underpins your study and practice, and allows you to fulfil your role in an ethical and principled manner is essential.

It is not within the remit of this text to outline all the legislation that informs every level of your practice to ensure that you are an accountable practitioner, competent to practise as a nursing associate. Other books are available for this, some of which you can find in the further reading section at the end of this chapter. However, knowledge of key Acts of Parliament is essential to your understanding of safe medicines administration in conjunction with the standards imposed on nursing associates by the Nursing and Midwifery Council contained in *The Code: Professional Standards of practice and behaviour for nurses, midwives and nursing associates* (NMC, 2018b).

The Nursing and Midwifery Council exists to safeguard the health and well-being of the public and it does this in several ways. It describes educational requirements for the health professionals it monitors, dictating what aspects of care must be included within any higher education establishment's curriculum for degrees, foundation degrees and apprenticeship pathways. For nursing associates, it describes expectations within its standards of proficiency, as seen at the beginning of each of this book's chapters relating to medicines management. The NMC publishes standards for registrants to uphold and acts to ensure that these standards are adhered to by use of disciplinary hearings and sanctions; they therefore act as assurance of your professional integrity. It also publishes guidance and standards that act as a resource.

If studying as an apprentice, the Institute for Apprenticeships and Technical Education (2022) sets out the skills and knowledge you will need to demonstrate in order to obtain an accredited award from your higher education institute. If undertaking this route, your programme of study will have been approved by the NMC and will include the occupational duties, knowledge, skills and behaviours that you will need to understand and be able to demonstrate. These, including the principles of medicines management, are taken from the *Nursing Associate Curriculum Framework* developed by Higher Education England

(HEE, 2016). HEE is an organisation that exists specifically to support the delivery of excellent healthcare and health improvement. Its remit is to ensure that the workforce has the right skills, values and behaviours to fulfil healthcare needs.

Accountability and responsibility

The Nursing and Midwifery Council states in its *Code: all professionals we regulate exercise professional judgement and are accountable for their work* (NMC, 2018b, p4), which shows just how fundamental to your practice the concepts of accountability and responsibility are, and how professionalism is key to upholding these. They are particularly important when considering the safe administration of medicines, so it is important that you understand exactly what these terms mean.

Accountability requires you to explain your actions or omissions to individuals to whom you owe a duty. This may be the duty of care to your patient, your obligation to your employer, a professional or a legal duty. This accountability is how you justify your actions to others.

Responsibility is the sense of ownership for the quality of your actions. As a nursing associate, you will need to decide in what way you practise and what interventions are in the best interests of your patients. You will have the responsibility to reflect on your practice and to continue to develop to ensure you are giving the highest standard of care possible.

Vicarious liability is another important concept to understand in relation to safe patient care, including medicines management. This legal principle protects employees from individual litigation. This is because employers are liable for the acts of their employees. This means that aggrieved patients or their carers may sue the organisation rather than individual healthcare workers if something untoward happens. It is important to note that this protection is only provided if employees are working within their normal duties and if they do not commit a criminal offence. It is quite acceptable for you as a nursing associate to be involved in medicines administration and your organisation should support you if an untoward event occurs. In contrast, you could not expect your employer to support your actions if you were undertaking surgery, for example, as it is not a normal part of your role. It is important to emphasise that this protection awarded by employers is dependent upon trainee and registered nursing associates working within their employing organisation's definitions of the role and scope of practice, and this may vary from organisation to organisation and over time. Your employer has a responsibility to oversee your role through governance structures, and if they expect medicines administration which is not documented within the NMC *standards of proficiency*, they will need to **mitigate against** potential risk by using locally agreed education, training, policy and protocols (HEE, 2017). Therefore, as with all professional registrants, there is a requirement that you keep up to date with changing local policy and procedures.

Understanding the theory: Accountability and responsibility

While the theory of accountability, responsibility and vicarious liability may seem complex when you first consider it, it can be quite simple and something you have been

(Continued)

(Continued)

doing already in your daily practice. Any time you have cared for a service user to the best of your ability, making sure you did so in line with your organisation's guidance on how the care should be done, you have demonstrated accountability and responsibility, and have enjoyed the protection from your employer. This is an example of you putting the theory into practice.

The purpose of accountability and responsibility is to ensure that the public and patients are not harmed by the things you do or by those you fail to do. In order to provide maximum protection, four areas of law are drawn together to hold you to account. You can be held to account by the patient, through **tort law**, through your employer, through your contract of employment, through your professional body via the Nursing and Midwifery order 2001 (HMSO, 2002) and by societal law. Society holds you to account through public law derived from Acts of Parliament, and breaching these may attract a criminal charge and possibly a custodial sentence. Therefore, it is important to have a good understanding of these and what they mean to you.

The Medicines Act 1968

In the United Kingdom, the Medicines Act 1968, in conjunction with European legislation, governs the production and supply of medications. This includes the control of each stage of manufacture and distribution including import and export. Each stage is subject to licensing arrangements and requires a marketing authorisation, previously called a product licence. These authorisations are administered and monitored by the Medicines and Healthcare products Regulatory Agency (MHRA) whose role is to regulate the clinical, cost-effective and safe use of medicines to ensure that patients get the maximum benefit from the medicines they need, while at the same time minimising potential harm (MHRA, 2022). This marketing authorisation specifies the uses for which the medicinal product is licensed. As more evidence from constant use becomes available, the drug companies can ask the MHRA for new indications to be added to the authorisation, if a product is found to have additional benefits that it was not originally developed for. An example might be aspirin, which is useful as an analgesic for mild pain and at a lower dose used as an antiplatelet drug. If a product does not have authorisation, it is described as **unlicensed**. If used outside the terms of its authorisation, it is described as **off-licence**. Prescribers who wish to use unlicensed or off-licence medications do so under their own responsibility. The General Medical Council (GMC) gives doctors very specific guidelines, as does the NMC for nurses and General Pharmaceutical Council (GPhC) for pharmacist prescribers, when prescribing unlicensed medicines; they may be used when no suitable licensed medicine meets the patient's needs. This may include the use of a medicine for a child that was not specifically developed for children. It may include when a licensed medicine is not available in the format required – for example, a tablet form of a medicine may have a licence, but the syrup form of this same medicine may not. It may include the use of imported medications or those still undergoing clinical trial. The *British National Formulary* (BNF) denotes these medications with a black triangle symbol and, if involved in administration, you will need to understand your responsibility for monitoring and reporting of adverse effects. This will be discussed further in Chapter 4.

It is also important to be aware that there are pharmacological and legal implications for altering medications. Drugs only have a licence to be administered in the form in which they are packaged. Crushing a tablet or opening a capsule for ease of administration will affect the kinetics and dynamics of the medication. In other words, the drug may be absorbed faster or slower than intended or have a different therapeutic effect. This means that the product will fall outside its specific marketing authorisation or licence. As a nursing associate, while this may seem a kindness to assist a service user to take their medicines, you need to be aware that this act means that you will be liable for any adverse effects caused by this misadministration. In cases such as these, it is always advisable to seek advice from the pharmacist for efficacy and alternatives.

The Medicines Act 1968 divides medicinal products into three groups for the purpose of supply (HMSO, 1968).

- **Prescription-only medicines (POMs)** can only be sold or supplied when there is a prescription written that authorises the transaction. Most drugs encountered in healthcare are POMs. This group of medicinal products are highly regulated by law which dictate what constitutes a prescription, who is authorised to handle the medicinal product, the storage and the documentation which must be kept regarding all aspects of the transaction. There are three classes of POMs: those that contain a listed substance, those products that are for parenteral use, these being medicines administered by a route other than the mouth and alimentary canal and those containing a drug that may be subject to misuse. There are additional restrictions or controls on the use of drugs that may be subject to misuse and these are known therefore as **controlled drugs (CDs)**.
- **Pharmacy medicines (P-medicines)** can only be sold by a pharmacist or under the supervision of a pharmacist from a registered pharmacy premises. These are often lower-strength POMs intended for short-term use. Patients can consult with the pharmacist regarding symptoms and appropriate treatments.
- **General sales list medicines (GSLs)** are those products with the lowest level of control over their sale and supply. They can be sold from any lockable outlet. They can only be sold in their original packaging, and there are limitations on the labelling, strength and packet size. These medicinal products are considered safe for people to buy without professional healthcare advice.

The Medicines Act 1968 additionally specifies the **labelling** requirements of medications. These labels must be clearly written in English and must be legible, clear and comprehensive (HMSO, 1968). For safety, medicines should not be stored outside of this original container. The label will contain the product name, the pharmaceutical form, such as a tablet or oral syrup, the strength of the active and non-active ingredients – for instance, the preservatives in eye drops and the quantity of liquid or number of tablets within the container. In addition, the labelling must include the expiry date, specific storage requirements – for example, if a medication needs to be stored at a specific temperature, the drug company name and the authorisation to sell number, the unique batch number, instructions for use and instructions for disposal. Medicines dispensed by a pharmacist will have additional labelling, including the patient's details, and the dispenser will ensure that appropriate information leaflets accompany each medication.

Now that you have discovered that medications have different classifications, complete Activity 1.2 in order to test your understanding

Activity 1.2   Critical thinking

You are asked by a friend for some advice regarding their persistent migraines and associated nausea. Use the *British National Formulary* (BNF) to assign the following medicines as prescription only (POM), pharmacy only (P), general sales list (GSLs) or controlled drug (CD):

- Sumatriptan (Imigran) 50mg tablets for migraine relief
- Box of 32 paracetamol 500mg tablets for symptom relief
- Buprenorphine 5 (BuTrans) patch for pain relief
- Box of 16 ibuprofen 200mg for symptom relief
- Propanolol 80 mg tablets for symptom control
- Box of 8 prochlorperazine 3mg (Buccastem) tablets for nausea

What advice might you give as a nursing associate?

An outline answer is given at the end of this chapter.

Now that we have reviewed the different classifications of medicines, as described in the Medicines Act 1968, we can explore other laws that dictate aspects of medicine management in practice.

The Misuse of Drugs Act 1971

In recognition of the danger to health that some drugs represented, the Dangerous Drugs Act 1920 restricted possession and prescribing, and implemented penalties for improper use of certain addictive products. With the advent of the Medicines Act in 1968, revision was required to reflect the new legal framework and required these dangerous drugs to be divided into **schedules and classes**. The potential for the misuse of these drugs gave rise to legislation that added levels of control to their use. The Misuse of Drugs Act 1971; HMSO 1971) was initiated to prevent the misuse of CDs by placing restrictions on the manufacture, import, possession, supply and export dependent on their schedule, with the classes A, B and C and a temporary class relating to the penalties imposed for misuse. Class A drugs are subject to the highest penalties and class C the lowest. The temporary class allows restrictions to be applied to new, so-called designer drugs, in a timely manner as they appear on the scene.

The Misuse of Drugs Regulations 2001 and Controlled Drugs (Supervision of management & use) Regulations 2013

These regulations govern the use of CDs in practice environments. Each CD is allocated to one of five schedules according to the level of control exercised over it. Each category represents the therapeutic use of the drug and its potential for misuse (HMSO, 2001, 2013) (see Table 1.1).

Table 1.1   The five schedules of controlled drugs

Schedule 1	Limited official medical use – e.g. LSD, cannabis, ecstasy	Possession and supply prohibited unless under Home Office rule
Schedule 2	Includes the opiates – e.g. morphine	Full controlled drug restriction – register required
Schedule 3	Synthetic opiates – e.g. barbiturates	Specific prescription requirements
Schedule 4	Certain benzodiazepines, anabolic steroids	Minimal control, records required
Schedule 5	Lower strength codeine	Minimal control, less stringent documentation

Misuse of drugs (designation) Order 2018 Amendment

In November 2018 (Home Office Circular, 2018), a statutory order was implemented to amend the 2001 Misuse of Drugs Regulations. This allows a legal route for cannabis-based products to be prescribed by doctors on the GMC specialist register in strictly controlled circumstances. The 2018 regulations define *cannabis-based products for medicinal use in humans* and rescheduled them as a Schedule 2 medicine. Only products defined will be rescheduled; any other product containing cannabis or its resin, cannabinol or its derivatives remain a Schedule 1 drug with possession and supply prohibited. The amendment does not impact on the offence of cultivation of the cannabis plant, or offences relating to recreational use, and this remains a class B CD and subject to associated penalties.

To support specialist clinicians' decisions to prescribe, the **National Institute for Health and Care Excellence (NICE, 2021)** has produced clinical guidelines for these unlicensed medicinal products. These are now available at www.nice.org.uk/guidance/ng144. Further information is obtainable for service users and healthcare professionals from MHRA, Royal College of Physicians guidance and NHS England.

Activity 1.3 will now explore the use of cannabis further in relation to providing patient care.

Activity 1.3   Critical thinking

Go back and review Mary's case study at the beginning of this chapter. Using the questions below, consider the implications of Mary confiding her use of cannabis to control her early multiple sclerosis symptoms.

- Which schedule or level of control does cannabis have?
- Are there any safeguarding concerns raised with this case study?
- As a nursing associate, how could you address her disclosure of cannabis use and support her in relation to her anxiety and panic attacks?

An outline answer is given at the end of this chapter.

Having reviewed the levels of control required for medicines that may be subject to misuse, we can explore other laws that affect how we manage medicines in practice.

The Health Act 2006 (updated in 2009)

Within practice, healthcare workers will be governed by **standard operating procedures (SOPs)** as required by the Health Act 2006; HMSO, 2006). These documents explain the procedures, accountability and responsibilities of employers when dealing with CDs. These tighter controls came as a direct consequence of the *Safeguarding patients reports*, outlining lessons learnt from the Dr Shipman case (HSMO, 2007).

Each employer is required to appoint an **accountable officer**, someone who does not ordinarily handle CDs within the organisation and who reports to the board, and suitably appointed individuals to witness the destruction of CDs. Prescribing and requisitioning must be monitored, including the validity and duration of prescriptions. With the **Care Quality Commission** (CQC, 2022a) recommending the use of a standard CD requisition form, appropriate storage, restricted access, secure transport, accurate documentation and formal escalation procedures need to be identified and followed.

Within your organisation, the standard operating procedures will specify who can order CDs, the process to follow, who can transport them and the designated personnel who can receive and enter the receipt into the CD register. This may differ from organisation to organisation and, as a nursing associate, you need to be familiar with your workplace requirements.

You will find in your organisation that CDs are stored in a particular way, with a locked cupboard within another locked cupboard. The keys for both are kept separate and warning lights allow practice areas to know when the cupboards are being accessed. A drug register of the cupboard's contents is kept and all administration, including patients' names and doses, are recorded. When administering a CD, a procedure must be followed, and local policies will dictate who may be involved at each level of the management of the CDs within the organisation. As a nursing associate, you will need to check local policy arrangements as they may differ from organisation to organisation. Activity 1.4 explores this further. In community settings, service users will require advice to maintain safe and appropriate home storage.

Activity 1.4   Work-based learning

Review your organisation's policy on the use and administration of CDs. Some areas of practice may place extra checks to ensure safe usage.

As this answer is based on your own observation, there is no outline answer at the end of this chapter.

Now that you have reviewed your organisation's policies for the use and administration of CDs, as described by the Health Act 2006, we can explore other laws that influence medicines management in practice.

The Human Medicines Regulations 2012

In August 2012, the Human Medicines Regulations (HMSO, 2012) came into force, simplifying much of the medicines management legislation and incorporating European Union legislation on monitoring the safety of medicines. It introduced changes to reflect modern medicines management. Under these regulations, POMs can only be given in accordance with the directions of the prescriber for the named patient. However, these regulations include exemptions for certain groups of registered health professionals to supply or administer certain medicines on their own initiative. An example of this would be paramedics treating acutely unwell or injured people. These regulations also list certain Schedule 19 medicines that may be administered by anyone for the purpose of saving a life in an emergency – for example, adrenaline 1:1,000 up to 1 mg for intramuscular use in anaphylaxis, as can be found in autoinjectors) (see Chapter 4 regarding anaphylaxis causes and treatment). Glucose, glucagon and hydrocortisone injections as well as snake venom antiserum are also currently included within this list. Individual employers may have local protocols in place to support healthcare professionals covered under Schedule 19 and may provide dosing instructions and define the circumstances in which medication should be administered (HEE, 2017).

In addition to specific medicines-related legislation, there are other laws that will have an impact on medicines optimisation, and you will need to have a knowledge of, and be able to apply, the requirements of these to fulfil your nursing associate duties. Table 1.2 includes some of these Acts and the consideration needed in relation to medicines management.

Table 1.2   Associated medicines management consideration for some more general laws

Name of statute	Medicines management consideration
The Mental Health Act 1983/ Amendment 2007; HMSO, 1983, 2007	Centres on entry into, care within and discharge from institutions. Strengthens rights of patients under compulsory powers.
	Detention does not necessarily mean compulsory treatment.
	Requires an understanding of the concepts of consent and covert administration for medicines management.
The Mental Capacity Act 2005/ Amendment 2019; HMSO, 2005, 2019	Designed to protect individuals who cannot make decisions for themselves, based on five key principles.
	Requires an understanding of the concepts of consent and covert administration for medicines management.
General Data Protection (GDP) Act 2018 HMSO (2018)	Identifies the need to follow data protection principles that include timely, accurate, appropriate and secure record-keeping when administering medicines.

(Continued)

Table 1.2   (Continued)

Name of statute	Medicines management consideration
The Children's Act 2004; HMSO, 2004	Protects the interests of children and young people.
	Requirement for safety, dignity, privacy and comfort when administering medicines.
The Care Act 2014; HMSO, 2014a	Highlights the principles of person-centred approach for safeguarding vulnerable adults.
	Requirement for safety, dignity, privacy and comfort when administering medicines.
Disability Discrimination Act 1995; Equality Act 2010; HMSO, 1995, 2010	Identifies the requirement to make reasonable adjustments to ensure equality of access to healthcare.
	May require solutions to medicines administration concerns – for example, associated with poor dexterity or reduced sight.
	Requirement for safety, dignity, privacy and comfort when administering medicines.

Many of these considerations will be discussed further in Chapter 4 which explores the procedures for the safe administration of medicines to different client groups. However, it is essential to discuss two further pieces of legislation here when considering our service users' safety.

Health and Safety Act 1974

Safety of ourselves and our patients is paramount in healthcare. The responsibilities of employers and the duties owed by employees are described within the Health and Safety Act 1974; HMSO, 1974 and its supplementary regulations and orders. Healthcare organisations will have policies and procedures for the practice environment you are working in with recommendations for the use of hand hygiene, personal protective equipment, the safe use and disposal of sharps and the disposal of hazardous waste.

Reporting accidents and incidents within practice is an essential component of monitoring the effectiveness of health and safety measures. There is a legal requirement to report certain accidents to the Health and Safety Executive, while others will require local reporting measures. Your practice areas will require the reporting of dangerous occurrences.

Hospitals are dangerous places, with patients suffering complex health and social care problems that require powerful modern treatments in a pressured and demanding environment. In the NHS, it is believed that a critical incident occurs in up to 10 per cent of all hospital admissions – that is, about 850,000 adverse events a year and at the cost of billions of pounds and untold human suffering. While human error is inevitable, sadly the same mistakes can happen time and time again with unsafe practices and procedures, and poor equipment usage. In order to minimise risk and to make practice areas safer, managers need personnel to report all instances of dangerous occurrences. Safety is the responsibility of all staff and organisations need to foster an environment where safety is the priority rather than concern for individual blame. In order to do this, many organisations have lowered the threshold for reporting, so that even minor incidents or near-misses are reported. **Near-misses** are events that might have resulted in harm but, due to a timely intervention by healthcare providers or the patient or their family, did not result in injury. As well as reporting minor events, your organisation will require scrutiny of **serious adverse events**. These are described as any unfavourable and unintended sign, including abnormal laboratory results, symptoms or a disease associated with treatment. In human drug trials, they are defined as any untoward medical occurrence that results in hospitalisation or causes the extension of hospitalisation, an event which is life threatening or results in death. **Never events** are serious, largely preventable patient safety incidents that should not occur if healthcare providers have implemented national guidance. From NHS data, between April 2020 and March 2021 187,670 medication incidents were reported in England, with 112 of these causing severe harm and 58 resulting in death (NHS England, 2021). Your organisation will have local guidance for these **critical and major incidents**, and you will need to refer to your local policies for definitions and reporting mechanisms.

Health and Social Care Act 2008; Regulations 2014

This Bill (HMSO, 2014b) seeks to enhance professional regulation and created the CQC to focus on providing assurance about the safety and quality of care for patients and service users with some aspects relating specifically to medicines management. This surveillance includes scrutiny of both organisations and individuals through governance. **Clinical governance** is defined as *a system through which NHS organisations are accountable for continuously improving the quality of their services and safeguarding high standards of care by creating an environment in which excellence in clinical care will flourish* (Scally and Donaldson, 1998, p61). It is the system for reviewing standards, errors and failings in order to learn and make improvements. It requires an organisation to have a culture of seeking out areas of good practice and championing them, and areas of poorer practice and improving upon them. For you as a nursing associate, it will involve ensuring that you have the knowledge and skills to undertake specific care, known as your **competence**, and recognising and addressing your limitations, as well as being involved in aspects of **clinical audit** to collate and examine information about care within your organisation. A common form of audit in medicines management is the collection of prescribing data to allow organisations to review and compare prescribing practices. **Risk management** is an important aspect of clinical governance. It recognises that organisations have a duty of care to their service users by ensuring that employees work to a set of minimum standards governed by the organisation's policies and procedures. If incidents and errors occur, including those involving medicines administration, the NMC and CQC highlight the importance of an open culture or **duty of candour** (CQC, 2015; NMC, 2022) with the intention that healthcare providers are open and honest with their service users. In this way, patients should receive truthful information, reasonable support and an apology as necessary.

Activity 1.5 asks you to reflect on safety in healthcare environments and to consider an event where harm may have come to a service user due to poor medicines management.

Activity 1.5   Reflection

Think of an example when you have seen, heard of or been involved in a mistake involving medicines administration. Consider the following questions.

*   What happened?
*   How was it discovered?
*   Who was involved?
*   How was it reported?
*   How was it investigated and what were the outcomes?
*   How has practice changed or been improved as a result?

As this answer is based on your own observation and reflection, there is no outline answer at the end of this chapter.

You may wish to discuss this reflection with colleagues and retain the information in a personal portfolio.

Now that you have reflected on clinical governance and an individual's responsibility for risk management, you can reassure yourself that you not only understand the legal considerations associated with medicines administration but also can, in fact, put it into practice.

Understanding the theory: Legislation

At the beginning of this chapter, we stated that you were not training to be lawyers, and it may seem that there has been a lot of theory here for you to read and understand. We know that this theory can seem complex and daunting; however, you will already have been abiding by much of this legislation during your daily practice and in your home lives without being overtly aware of it. Any occasion when you have bought over-the-counter paracetamol, looked at the label on a medicine prescribed for you or a family member, and observed and been part of administration in the workplace that has followed local policies, you have been working within UK law. These are all examples of your putting theory into practice.

As well as the legal considerations which you have now explored, there is a requirement for you to understand the roles, responsibilities and scope of practice of other members of the interdisciplinary team in relation to medicines management.

Roles of the multidisciplinary team

As a nursing associate, your role requires the safe management and administration of medicines across the fields of nursing and the age continuum, and in a variety of practice settings.

As such, you will need to have an awareness of the roles of other members of the multidisciplinary team depending on your practice area, as well as understanding the terminology they use. Interprofessional or multidisciplinary team-working is essential in healthcare to ensure optimum care for the service users and is seen as a key factor in improving medicines management. However, the terms used in medicines management are often misunderstood and used interchangeably, so it is important that you develop a full understanding of the key terms, which we will now explore.

In relation to medicines management, **supply** relates to the giving of medicines to a service user for them to take away and take over a specified period and in a certain way. **Administration** describes the giving of a medication to a patient while you observe them taking it or assisting them with this process. **Prescribing** involves the selection of the appropriate medication by a recognised practitioner, and **dispensing** is the provision of this medication for the patient to take away. In all cases, the person undertaking any of these roles must be competent to do so.

Prescribers fall into two categories: medical prescribers, which include registered doctors and dentists, and **non-medical prescribers**. To prescribe a medicinal product, an individual must be registered with a professional body, like the General Medical Council, having first undertaken the relevant training, and have a licence to prescribe from the **formulary** associated with their qualification. Non-medical prescribers and their prescribing rights are described in the *Medicines Matters* document (NHS, 2018), which denotes the relevant formulary that is linked to their recordable qualification and their accountability under their professional codes of conduct. **Independent prescribers** can prescribe any licensed medicine and unlicensed medicines that are within their formulary provided they have assessed the patient, diagnosed and have a strong rationale for medication choice, as well as ensuring they are working within their level of competence and their organisation's policies and procedures. **Supplementary prescribing** is a voluntary partnership between the patient, a non-medical prescriber and an independent prescriber who must be a doctor or a dentist. In these circumstances, a **clinical management plan (CMP)** is agreed that allows for the ongoing prescribing support of patients with long-term conditions. All prescribers are accountable under their professional codes and ethics for their prescribing decisions, actions and omissions (RPS, 2023).

Prescriptions do not follow a single format in healthcare settings, so you will need to familiarise yourself with the documentation of the organisation you are working for. Medicine is prescribed for a specific individual as a written instruction as a **patient-specific direction** and will include the dose, route and frequency of a medicine or appliance. This document is patient-specific and the drugs dispensed to fulfil the order are the property of the named individual. The prescription form is a legal document and is classified as **secure stationery**. Tight controls exist to regulate the ordering of prescription pads (FP10), their storage, use and disposal. **Patient group directions (PGDs)** exist to allow certain professional groups, identified in the direction, to administer drugs in line with strict criteria and instructions laid out in the directive to groups of individuals clearly defined in the document. As a nursing associate, you will administer medications through patient-specific directions, but not through the patient group direction. However, as with all aspects of your practice, you will need to refer to your own organisation's policies and procedures, as your ability to administer under a patient group direction may change in the future.

When dealing with prescriptions, you need to remember your own level of personal accountability and responsibility. Just because a member of the interprofessional team has prescribed a medication, as a registered nursing associate you must satisfy yourself that the prescription has been correctly written, is legible and appropriate prior to any administration. Any concerns should be immediately brought to the attention of the prescriber. The safe administration of all medicines will be discussed further in Chapter 4.

Pharmacists play a key role in the safe management of medications. Their specialist knowledge, skill and precision are required to prepare and dispense medications safely. They are experts in medicines and their use, and as such are a very valuable resource to you as a nursing associate. They can offer advice and support on types of medicines, side effects, dosages, contraindications and alternatives as appropriate. They can also be called upon to be the first port of call for service users requesting symptom control and healthcare advice.

Increasingly, pharmacists within secondary care settings use a **one-stop dispensing** system to improve medicines management safety and reduce waste. Traditionally, patients surrendered the medicines they were taking prior to admission to hospital staff, and fresh supplies were dispensed and used throughout their hospital stay. Then, on discharge, a new set of medications was dispensed and packaged for the service user to take out (TTO). As the patient's property, the original medications were also relinquished, if they had not been destroyed. One-stop dispensing allows the patient to receive a supply of medication in their name for their inpatient stay and, after checking, these then form the medications they will take home. This has the capacity to save money, but more importantly reduces the risk of patients taking both original and additional medicines together once at home.

As a nursing associate, you will inevitably work with other nurses and disciplines. Nursing registrants will work within their individual scope of practice and in adherence to their codes of practice (NMC, 2018b). Like you, they will adhere to *standards for administration of medication* (RPS, 2023) and employers' policies and procedures. As you will be working closely alongside these colleagues, as well as other professionals who may be supplementary pre-scribers, like dieticians, for example, you will need to clearly understand all aspects of both their and your competence, accountability and responsibility.

Other healthcare staff play their part in ensuring the safety of medicines administration. In some instances, healthcare assistants may be delegated responsibility of administering med-icines in certain settings, if deemed appropriate by the registered nurse, who is ultimately responsible. Other important tasks involving non-qualified members of the multidisciplinary team can include maintaining the cleanliness of practice areas, as well as safe transportation and disposal of medicine.

As stated at the beginning of this chapter, having a legal awareness that underpins your practice is essential, and throughout your nursing associate career new Legislation and amendments will be introduced. As an example, since the publication of the first edition of this text, the COVID-19 pandemic necessitated a response from the UK Government to cope with the volume of immunisations which needed to be administered and to support prescribers and vaccinators. A number of amendments to Legislation were produced. The Human Medicines (Coronavirus and Influenza) (Amendment) Regulations 2020 covered temporary author-isations for the vaccines, including the civil liability and immunity for participants in vacci-nation programmes and supported the expansion of the healthcare workforce who could administer. A later 2022 amendment was also made, which governs the arrangements for licensing, manufacture, wholesale dealing and supply. In addition, The National Health Service (Performers Lists, Coronavirus) (England) Amendment Regulations 2021 removed the requirement for medical practitioners to be on the performers list to deliver the COVID vaccine. It is clear therefore that a commitment to remaining up to date with current gover-nance requirements is essential for your professional practice.

This chapter has asked you to explore several considerations in relation to the legal and professional rationales for medicines management. Activity 1.6 asks you to reflect on what you have read and to check your understanding of the key concepts discussed.

Activity 1.6   Reflection

Now that you have worked through the chapter, consider the following questions.

- How can you define accountability for nursing associates?
- What is your role in the management of CDs?
- How do you report a clinical incident in your organisation?
- Can you describe the roles and responsibilities of the interprofessional team in relation to medicines management?

There are no sample answers to these questions. Where you are not confident in your knowledge of a topic, you may find it necessary to reread sections of this chapter or view the further reading and websites listed at the end of this chapter to assist you. Information for question 1 can be found in the accountability and responsibility section; question 2 in the Misuse of Drugs Act 1971 and the Misuse of Drugs regulations 2001 section; question 3 in the Health and Safety Act 1974 section and Question 4 in the last section of this chapter.

Now that you have had a chance to reflect on the contents of this chapter, you can see from the following summary that you have, in fact, explored a large amount of theory and been able to link this to your own practice.

Chapter summary

As you can see from this chapter, health professionals have various legal responsibilities for medicines management. This chapter has outlined the key legislation relating to medicines, including the Medicines Act 1968, the Misuse of Drugs Act 1971, and Misuse regulations 2001, the Health Act 2006; Human Medicines Regulations 2012, as well as other pertinent Acts of Parliament, which will ensure both ethical, professional and accountable medicines administration. It has defined the term 'controlled drug' and outlined the schedules and the standard operating procedures relating to the accountability, storage, administration, documentation and disposal of these medications.

The meaning of accountability, responsibility and vicarious liability, and the roles and responsibilities of the nursing associates and other members of the healthcare team in medicines administration has been described. This chapter has also discussed improving safety and the quality of care. It will have enabled you to understand the principles of health and safety, how to report risks and implement actions accordingly, and has outlined what constitutes a near-miss, a serious adverse event, a critical incident and a major incident.

The activities included in this chapter have invited you to consider what a medicine is, how these medicines are available, what your role is in acting as a resource to service users, what your organisation's policies and procedures are and how we can all work together to ensure safe and appropriate medicines management. This safe administration will be discussed further in Chapter 4.

Activities: Brief outline answers

Activity 1.1 Critical thinking (page 7)

The term 'medicine' describes any substance or combination of substances presented as having the properties of preventing or treating disease in human beings; or any substance or combination of substances that may be used by or administered to human beings with a view to restoring, correcting or modifying a physiological function by exerting a pharmacological, immunological or metabolic action, or making a medical diagnosis. A product may also be defined as something else, such as a cosmetic or health food, and that we need to consider the patient's perspective.

Activity 1.2 Critical thinking (page 11)

- Sumatriptan (Imigran) 50 mg tablets – POM
- Box of 32 Paracetamol 500mg tablets – P
- Buprenorphine 5 (BuTrans) patch – CD
- Box of 16 ibuprofen 200mg – GSL
- Propanolol 80 mg tablets – POM
- Box of 8 Prochlorperazine 3 mg (Buccastem) tablets – P

As a nursing associate, you can inform your friend of the availability and types of medications within your level of competence and knowledge. However, best practice would always be to advise your friend to seek urgent medical attention for persistent headaches to ensure the diagnosis of migraine and that it is nothing more sinister.

Activity 1.3 Critical thinking (page 13)

Cannabis is a Schedule 1 CD unless prescribed as a recognised cannabis-based product (NICE, 2021) and as such has class B penalties imposed for its misuse. The 2018 regulations continue to prohibit smoking of cannabis regardless of intentions.

Mary has a child and has disclosed being under the influence of an illicit drug. This would need to be explored further in a sensitive way to identify if there were safeguarding concerns in relation to her child. Clear documentation around these discussions is essential as well as honesty and transparency when making any referrals or escalation to social care/safe guarding team.

Professional accountability and integrity are needed in relation to Mary's disclosure about illicit drug use. As a nursing associate, you can listen and support her in a non-judgemental manner. A very brief intervention may be appropriate to support behaviour change in relation to her current cannabis use. NICE (2014) recommends ask, advise, assist. This may include advice around the risks associated with illicit drug use including the harmful affect it can have on physical and mental health, including potentially making her anxiety worse (Royal College of Psychiatrists, 2022), as well as interactions it may have on her prescribed medication. Assistance may involve referral to other professionals to seek alternative non-pharmacological treatments such as talking therapies or prescribed medication for her anxiety.

Further reading

To better understand accountability, responsibility and your position as a nursing associate with medicines management, the following titles may be helpful.

Brack, G, Franklin, P and Caldwell, J (2013) *Medicines Management for Nursing Practice.* Oxford: Oxford University Press.

Chapter 1 in this text will assist you to understand legal, professional and clinical boundaries relating to accountability and responsibility, and how to apply these to the administration and supply of medicines. It also explains major legislation relating to medicines.

Griffith, R Tengnah, C (2023) *Law and Professional Issues in Nursing* (6th edn). Exeter: SAGE.

This text provides conditions from which we can pursue our personal and professional lives, safeguarding our service users. It includes where laws come from and how legislation influences healthcare, ensuring protection of the vulnerable and ourselves.

Nursing and Midwifery Council (2018) *Standards of Proficiency for Nursing Associates.* London: NMC.

This document explains what is expected of nursing associates with regard to their professional conduct.

Useful websites

The following websites are useful resources to aid your understanding.

BNF Publications: www.bnf.org

This website allows you to search for specific medicines information and guides for medicines management.

Care Quality Commission: www.cqc.org.uk

This is the website for the independent regulator of health and social care services in England.

The official home of UK legislation: www.legislation.gov.uk

This website publishes a variety of legislation related to many different aspects of the law, including medicines management.

Medicines and Healthcare products Regulatory Agency: www.mhra.gov.uk

This website provides information on the role of the Medicines and Healthcare products Regulatory Agency, which ensures that medicines and medicinal products are safe to use.

National Institute for Health and Clinical Excellence: www.nice.org.uk

This website offers insights into prescribing practices and approved treatment regimes.

Nursing and Midwifery Council: www.nmc-uk.org

This website will allow you to further understand your professional and ethical responsibilities regarding medicine management.

Royal College of Nursing: www.rcn.org.uk

The membership organisation of over 435,000 nurses, midwives, healthcare assistants and nursing students.

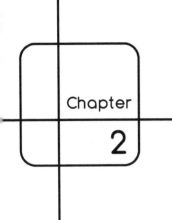

The human body, ageing and the disease process

Chapter aims

After reading this chapter, you will be able to:

- understand the basic integrated anatomy and physiology of body systems necessary to ensure homoeostasis and the impact medicines management has on this;
- gain an understanding of the body systems that relate directly to how medication is processed in the body;
- appreciate the effects of disease and ageing processes on the human body, and associated signs and symptoms that affect our service users and its implications for medicines management.

Introduction

You are visiting your friend's house when she informs you that her daughter Aashna, who is six months old, appears to have contracted a cold from her older brother. Your friend does not wish to trouble her GP as this is just a common cold. Your friend knows you are a trainee nursing associate and asks you to explain how infections are spread, if there is anything she should worry about with Aashna still being an infant, and if there are any medications you can suggest to relieve her daughter's symptoms.

Aashna's case study is an example of the importance of understanding the basic principles of the function of the human body and the ageing processes, the causes and resultant signs and symptoms of disease and how medications work. To understand these processes, this chapter will set out the organisation and function of the human body. First, it describes the cell, the most basic structural unit of the human body and its role in ensuring homoeostasis. It does this in conjunction with the integrated body systems, including the transport and communication systems, both internal and external, which will be examined next. The chapter will then help you to understand the body systems with distinct roles in medicines management, including the digestive, renal, cardiovascular and integumentary systems. Then we will describe the process of ageing and its effect on these body systems, as well as introduce the concept of disease processes known as pathophysiology.

It is acknowledged that science – the biology and chemistry associated with the function of the human body – is daunting to many in health and social care settings. This book is not designed as an anatomy and physiology text. There are many sources that you can explore to further develop your knowledge and understanding in this area, some of which we have highlighted at the end of the chapter. Nevertheless, a knowledge of basic structure and function of the cell and integrated body systems will help you to understand the basic physiology of disease processes, associated signs and symptoms, and the subsequent therapeutic and toxic effects of medications given to relieve or treat.

Before we examine these principles in more detail, let us start with an activity to help you reflect on your current knowledge of the science of the organisation and function of the human body.

Activity 2.1   Critical thinking

- List the organ systems of the body.
- Note the main function of each system.
- List the component organs.

An outline answer is given at the end of this chapter.

Having reflected on your current knowledge of tissues, organs and body systems, let us look at some of these in more detail.

The body and its constituents

The most basic structural unit of living organisms is the **cell**. Cells are arranged into tissues and organs. Apart from red blood cells, each cell has a nucleus which contains the genetic material for reproduction and regulation. All cells have a cytoplasm which contains a variety of organelles and a plasma membrane, site of the action of most medications, which separates the fluid within, called **intracellular**, and the fluid outside, called **extracellular**. The cell membrane is essential for cell integrity, as well as many of the mechanisms for maintaining homoeostasis. Without plasma membrane integrity, the cell will die. This is useful for some antibiotics that attack the cell wall of certain bacteria, known as cell wall synthesis inhibitors (e.g. penicillins). Without the cell wall to protect them, the bacteria burst and die (Figure 2.1).

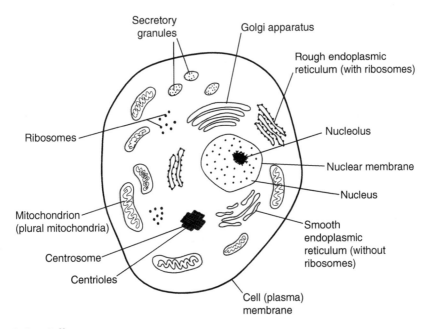

Figure 2.1   Cell structure

To maintain the stability of the cytoplasm, the fluid and its contents, within the plasma membrane requires **homoeostasis**. The internal environment of the cell is tightly controlled within narrow limits and requires several physiological mechanisms to maintain its constant state. Homoeostasis is maintained by control systems that detect and respond to changes in the internal environment and nearly all are regulated by negative feedback mechanisms. For instance, a drop in temperature triggers negative feedback that respond to the change in norm, activating mechanisms such as shivering and narrowing of blood vessels to rectify the situation. When the temperature normalises, mechanisms are deactivated so shivering stops and blood flow returns to normal.

As a function of homoeostasis, the plasma membrane acts as a selective barrier. It regulates what can pass into the cell and disposes of toxic waste products by both passive and active transport mechanisms, as well as providing channels or pores allowing the passage of small molecules. The plasma membrane also has embedded proteins, which have several functions. One type of protein located on the plasma membrane is the receptor which, when bound with specific chemicals such as hormones, chemical transmitters and medications, stimulate a reaction within the cell. Other plasma membrane proteins are surface antigens or genetically determined identifying markers. These allow the body to identify their own cells and recognise invaders or 'non-self' cells as part of the body's immune defence system.

The life cycle of the cell is dependent on the genetic make-up, which determines the rate at which each cell can multiply. Some cells multiply quickly, like those lining the gastrointestinal (GI) tract, while others reproduce more slowly. Although these timescales can be altered, hormones and chemicals can stimulate cell reproduction as required – for example, when the body requires more white blood cells when foreign proteins are identified as part of the body's immune response. Regardless of the rate of reproduction, each cell has approximately the same life cycle, consisting of the **interphase** when the cell grows and undertakes its normal activities and the **mitotic phase** when the cell divides and produces two identical daughter cells. Once a cell is damaged or useless, it can be harmful. **Apoptosis** is the rapid and irreversible process to efficiently eliminate these dysfunctional cells. A notable trait of cancer is the malignant cells' ability to avoid apoptosis, which allows tumour development.

Integrated body systems

In order for a person to fully function, their different cells, organs, tissues and body systems must work together as an integrated, interdependent whole. This requires the structures to be connected and effective transport and communication systems between all the different cell types. This has implications when one group of cells, organ or body system malfunctions, as it has an impact on other systems and parts of the body.

Transport systems include the cardiovascular system and lymphatic system. Within the cardiovascular system, blood transports essential substances throughout the body, including oxygen, nutrients and chemical substances, including medications and waste products. The lymphatic system, which begins as blind-ended tubes in the spaces between blood capillaries and tissue cells, known as the **interstitial space**, allows for the drainage of plasma protein, bacteria and cell debris into the bloodstream. It also contains lymph nodes situated at various points along the lymph vessels which filter lymph fluid, removing microbes and other materials, and provide the sites for formation and maturation of white blood cells.

Communication systems receive, collate and respond to information with both the internal and external environment. Internal communication involves mainly the nervous and endocrine system and is achieved in the human body using chemical messengers that act on the receptor of the target cell. These messengers include growth factors, hormones and neurotransmitters as signalling molecules. Most receptors are cell membrane proteins and they recognise signalling molecules like a lock recognising its key (see Chapter 3). The external communication involves the sensory nervous system.

The nervous system is a rapid communication system consisting of the brain, spinal cord and peripheral nerves, which either transmit signals from the body to the brain via sensory or afferent nerves, or transmit signals from the brain to an organ, such as a muscle, as a motor or efferent nerve. For example, when sensory nerves respond to pain on touching something sharp or hot, they trigger a motor response to move the hand away from the painful stimulus (see Figure 2.2). Communication along the nerve fibre is by an electrical impulse and these impulses or action potentials allow for rapid and fine adjustments to the body's function. Communication between nerve fibres requires the release of a chemical neurotransmitter which travels across the gap between the nerve cells to either stimulate or inhibit further action.

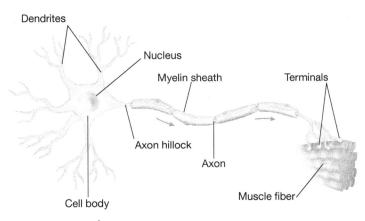

Figure 2.2   Action potential

Source: Gaskin (2019).

The endocrine system consists of a number of glands situated throughout the body. These glands make and secrete chemical messengers called hormones which, when circulated in the blood, influence cellular activity in the target tissues or organs. These hormones include insulin, glucagon, cortisol, testosterone and oestrogen. The endocrine glands respond to changes in the normal internal environment, and through negative feedback mechanisms control body functions in a slower and more precise manner than the fast-acting nervous control.

One further communication mechanism within the body is local signalling, which occurs between cells that are very close to each other; here a cell can initiate a response in an adjacent cell by the release of chemical messengers. This occurs, for example, with some cancers or as part of an inflammatory response where inflammatory mediators are released and act on the target mechanism of an adjacent cell initiating a local response, as well as entering the bloodstream and thus affecting other more distant target cells (Figure 2.3).

We need next to consider the body systems that are fundamental to our understanding of how medicines are processed within the body. Before we do this, review what you have learnt within this section by answering the following multiple-choice questions in Activity 2.2.

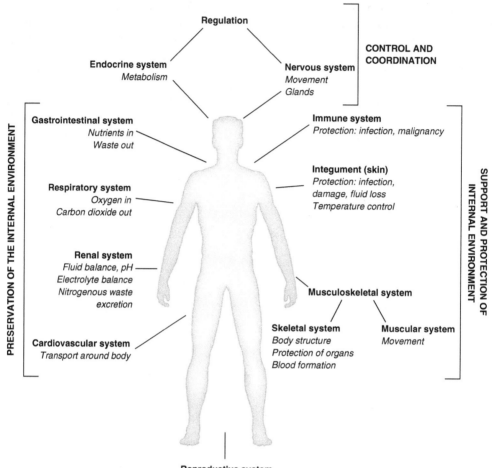

Figure 2.3 Body systems in homoeostasis (Rowe et al., 2023)

Activity 2.2   Critical thinking

1. The endocrine glands secrete:
   a) neurotransmitters;
   b) chemical transmitters called hormones;
   c) inflammatory mediators;
   d) electrical impulses.

2. The smallest living unit of the human body is:
   a) an organ;
   b) a tissue;

(Continued)

     c)   a cell;

     d)   an organ system.

3.   The regulation of body systems to maintain equilibrium is called:

     a)   transportation;

     b)   homoeostasis;

     c)   communication;

     d)   integration.

4.   Fluid found inside the cell membrane is called:

     a)   intracellular;

     b)   organelles;

     c)   interstitial;

     d)   extracellular.

An outline answer is given at the end of this chapter.

Having answered these questions and reviewed those areas you were uncertain of, let us consider how this physiology is organised in body systems to explain what happens to the medicines we administer.

Body systems with distinct roles in medicines management

While we acknowledge that human physiology requires all organs to work together as integrated, interdependent systems, there are certain organs and body systems that are fundamental for processing medication. This medication journey – how the body processes medication – involves absorption, distribution, metabolism and excretion, which will be explored further in the next chapter. Before we examine the body systems in more detail, take some time to reflect on your current knowledge of the digestive, hepatic and renal systems and the implications for medicines management. Activity 2.3 will help you with this.

Activity 2.3   Critical thinking

In Activity 2.1 you were asked to list the systems of the body, noting the organs involved and describing the system's main function. From this investigation, now consider the consumption of a roast dinner with a glass of wine. What path do the constituent parts of this meal take and what processes do they undergo?

An outline answer is given at the end of this chapter.

Now that you have reflected on how the food and drink you consume travels through the body, let us examine this in more detail.

The **digestive system's** main function is to ingest and digest food, absorb nutrients and eliminate any waste products. Medication via oral, enteral and rectal routes all travel along elements of the GI tract where they are absorbed into the bloodstream and distributed via the circulatory system.

There is a range of accessory organs to aid the digestive process, including salivary glands, the tongue and teeth to mechanically break down food and aid movement through the gut, known as gut motility. Gut motility also aids **mechanical digestion** through the contraction and relaxation of the gut, known as **peristalsis**. **Chemical digestion** occurs when enzymes are activated to break down contents, digesting proteins into smaller amino acids and fats into triglycerides to prepare for absorption. Oral medication can also be digested, loosing its potency, although medication capsules and coating can help prevent this, an example being the enteric coating of tablets like non-steroidal anti-inflammatory drugs such as naproxen. Not only does this coating increase the therapeutic effect of the drug it also helps prevent activation of the drug too early which can lead to stomach ulceration and irritation.

Once broken down, nutrients, except fats, are absorbed into the bloodstream through finger-like cells on the surface of the small intestine called villi. Fats enter the lymphatic system via the lacteals of the villi. Movement occurs through active transport, facilitated or passive diffusion, with this process being affected by the concentration gradient, the pH of the environment and solubility (see Chapter 3).

Most digestion and absorption happen in the small intestine, with nutrient-rich blood flowing from the intestine straight to the liver via the portal vein; this is how oral medication enters the liver. Contents that are not absorbed into the bloodstream continue down the GI tract through the large intestine, which contains healthy bacteria known as the gut microbiome. The large intestine has responsibility for reabsorbing water and salts. Fibre helps to combine unabsorbed contents and compact it, allowing excretion as faeces, as well as having important functions in protecting the microbiome that produces vitamins such as vitamin B12, thiamine and riboflavin.

Certain factors impair digestion and absorption; vomiting caused by distention or irritation to the stomach means that partially broken-down food, known as **chyme**, is ejected from the stomach, resulting in nutrients and medication not being digested. Diarrhoea does not allow optimal absorption and can remove the gut microbiome in the process. Similarly, adrenaline can also speed up the digestive process, which is why sometimes you need the toilet just before a stressful event. Digestive function matures from birth and diminishes with age. This causes drug absorption to be slower in newborns and infants. As a person ages, digestive function diminishes. Taste bud replacement lessens, rendering food less tasty and therefore less interesting. An inability or difficulty in swallowing, poorly fitting dentures or tooth loss and diminished chewing muscular strength can all render the mechanical breakdown of food difficult. In addition, there is an increasing risk of aspiration of food substances into the respiratory system with the resultant concerns this produces. The rate of peristalsis slows, increasing the risk of constipation and haemorrhoids, and the absorption rate slows. All these factors can lead to our elderly service users' suffering from loss of appetite and poor nutrition. Deficiencies in diet and altered hormone production can also affect the body's internal communication systems and affect how medication is processed (see Chapter 3). The ageing GI tract therefore will have an impact on the uptake of medicines, as well as potentially requiring medication to aid its function and to manage symptoms.

Other factors may impair the body's ability to digest and absorb medications. The body's pH can affect a medicine's ability to diffuse and distribute effectively through the body and certain foods can impair medication absorption. For example, tetracyclines, a type of antibiotic, cannot be taken with milk as they bind to the calcium in milk which prevents absorption in the gut. The unwanted effects of a medication can alter the normal GI tract physiology. For example, calcium channel blockers like nifedipine relax the smooth muscle of the heart to reduce blood pressure; this can also inadvertently relax smooth muscle in the gut and reduce its motility. Regular use of NSAIDs (non-steroidal anti-inflammatory drugs) like naproxen taken for musculoskeletal disorders is a risk factor for gastric ulcers, particularly in the older population (BNF, 2023). Stomach acid can cause the medication to diffuse into mucosal cells where they become trapped and cause damage to the lining of the stomach and thus affect digestion.

You may have observed other factors and conditions in your practice experience that will affect medication digestion and absorption. Activity 2.4 asks you to reflect and consider an example.

Activity 2.4   Reflection

Consider the impact of digestive disorders – for example, inflammatory bowel disease (IBD) on medicines management.

An outline answer is given at the end of this chapter.

Now that you have explored how food, drink and medicines are digested and absorbed, let us examine how the resultant components are processed within our bodies.

The **liver** acts as a processing, cleansing and production hub. How and when a medicine is processed affects its duration of action, its effectiveness and toxicity; therefore, the liver is an important organ in relation to medicines management.

The liver processes nutrients, turning them into useful components as well as detoxifying harmful substances in the blood through chemical breakdown, known as metabolism. For instance, it converts ammonia, a waste product from protein metabolism, into urea so that it can be excreted. It also metabolises other substances, including alcohol and medication. The process of metabolism reduces the therapeutic effect of a drug, meaning by this stage in the journey, that drug availability is significantly reduced, with on average only 10–20 per cent remaining. This process, known as **first pass metabolism**, will be explored further in Chapter 3. The liver also produces important substances, including 90 per cent of the body's plasma proteins. These include albumin, which plays an important role in medicines distribution, c-reactive protein and clotting factors. It also produces and secretes bile that is required for the breakdown of fat in the small intestine. It stores glycogen and is involved in glucose homoeostasis.

The liver's function in metabolism is also important for successful drug excretion. For instance, thiopental, a general anaesthetic, is an example of a drug that is converted from a lipid to water-soluble substance in the liver so that it can be excreted. The half-life, the time taken for half of the drug to be eliminated, of this medication when metabolised to become water soluble is around 10 hours; if it is not metabolised and remained lipid soluble, it would have a half-life of up to 25 years (EMC, n.d.).

Certain factors can impair metabolism. Inflammation of the liver, which can be caused by misuse of substances, viral infections and the accumulation of fat cause the liver to malfunction. In these situations, liver cells, known as hepatocytes, are unable to function and metabolise nutrients as normal. This causes drug metabolism to become impaired and therefore the potency of medication can be stronger and lead to toxicity. Infants are more prone to greater first pass metabolism due to increased hepatic clearance. Metabolism also becomes slower as we age, meaning detoxification of drugs is less effective, which needs to be considered when managing medications. This is the reason why many medications, particularly oral medications that are metabolised by the liver, are contraindicated or a lower dose is indicated in service users with hepatic impairment.

As well as the liver, the kidneys have an important role in medicine excretion. The renal system acts as one of our means of elimination by filtering the blood and ensuring that essential nutrients are reabsorbed and waste products are removed through urine. Homeostatic functions, including messages from hormones, allow the body to maintain an equilibrium in relation to fluid and electrolyte balance. This means that the urinary system works closely with the cardiovascular or circulatory system. A quarter of total cardiac output is delivered straight to the kidneys to enable them to function effectively. This means that medicines affecting one system may impact on the other. A good example of this is diuretic medication such as frusemide, commonly used to treat cardiac conditions such as heart failure by reducing oedema. This loop diuretic works at the loop of Henle within the kidneys inhibiting sodium reabsorption (EMC, n.d.). Water follows the unabsorbed sodium through osmosis, causing increased water loss as urination. This can affect fluid balance and a contraindication of frusemide is hypotension and hypovolaemia. Electrolyte balance can also be affected and requires monitoring. Hypokalaemia in particular is a risk factor with this medication.

As the urinary system is where much of our medication ends its journey and is excreted, it needs to be functioning fully for these drugs to be removed from the body at the appropriate time. Therefore, many medications are contraindicated in renal impairment, as there is the potential for them to circulate in the body longer than intended continuing to exert a pharmacological effect.

Renal function requires close monitoring in service users with long- or short-term kidney impairment, acute kidney injury or chronic kidney disease, as well as those who are on nephrotoxic medication such as gentamycin. Patients with heart disease, hypertension and diabetes are at high risk of developing kidney disease; in addition, these patients are commonly on numerous medications. If kidney function deteriorates, these medications are likely to cause adverse effects, with polypharmacy increasing the risk of this happening. If the renal function is impaired, electrolyte and fluid balance can also be affected.

Other factors can have an impact on medicine elimination. The pH of urine can impact on drug elimination. Whereas in the gut lipid-soluble drugs are more easily absorbed, water-soluble drugs are more easily excreted in urine. Most medicines are mildly acidic, and they will ionise to become more water-soluble if the urine is alkaline. This process is sometimes used in overdose situations in practice, changing the urine pH to speed up drug elimination.

The effectiveness of the urinary system varies across the ageing continuum. Clearance of a drug from the body is commonly reduced in neonates, particularly preterm infants, but this can become quicker than adults as children continue to grow. As a person ages the effectiveness of the urinary system diminishes. Kidney tissue decreases with the resultant loss of renal nephrons and reduced circulatory supply. The loss of muscle tone can affect both bladder function and urethra placement. For male service users, enlarged prostate glands can additionally impact on urinary flow and allow residual build-up of urine, resulting in increased risk of infection and associated symptoms. As with all medicines management, decreased organ and system function will have implications for prescribing, dosages and monitoring of service users and may require medicines to assist with function or relieve symptoms.

Having explored body systems that deal with nutrient processing, two further body systems need to be mentioned briefly as having an important role in medicines management, circulatory and integumentary. As identified earlier, the renal system works closely with the cardiovascular and circulatory system. The heart and blood vessels are essential for distribution around the body as well as having a distinct relationship with the lymphatic system to allow fluid drainage. Altered cardiovascular function will have implications for medicines management, as well as requiring specific medications to assist with function.

As with all body systems, ageing influences the circulatory system, although most of these changes are as a result of disease processes. The ability of the heart to pump effectively reduces cardiac output, cholesterol increases leading to thickened and less elastic blood vessels and the functional blood volume decreases. This reduced ability to distribute medicines, in addition to reduced blood supply to GI, liver and renal systems, will require altered prescribing, dosing and monitoring of service users when administering medicines.

The integumentary system is the body's first line of defence, with the skin functioning as the boundary between our bodies and the outside world. The skin, the largest organ of the body, assists with homeostasis by sensing change and having a role in maintaining equilibrium by regulation of heat and water loss.

You will have observed the function of the skin when administering subcutaneous, intramuscular and transdermal medicines and observing intravenous therapy. You will be aware from your practice areas, the concerns for healthcare professionals when this protective barrier is breached, and the specific care requirements to minimise potential harm from this. We will explore this later in this chapter when briefly describing our body's immune response and its links to medicines management.

You will additionally have observed as a person ages that their skin becomes more fragile, losing its elasticity, the capillary blood supply becomes more fragile, increasing the chance of bruising, and the skin becomes dry. Also, subcutaneous fat layers diminish, resulting in less insulation. This has implications for medicines administration in this age group, and you will be aware of the need to accommodate for these changes in your practice areas.

As a result of body systems working together, individuals can maintain health and resist disease. The **immune system** functions across all our body systems, infective agents such as bacteria, virus, fungus and parasites, known as **pathogens**, can enter through any orifice, as well as breaches in the skin. The first line of defence includes hostile environments for pathogens – for example, the acidity of urine and stomach contents, physiological barriers like the skin's integrity and fine hairs in the nose and bronchi known as cillia which can trap particles and allow mucus to remove them, as well as enzyme-rich fluids like saliva and tears which can break down pathogenic substances. The second line of defence is non-specific and allows engulfing cells, known as **phagocytes,** to destroy invading organisms. This is recognised in individuals by the infected area becoming swollen, painful and red due to increased blood flow and is described as **inflammation.**

The third line of defence is more specific and requires **lymphocytes** to respond to and destroy specific 'non-self' invaders. This response relies on the recognition of foreign proteins. Aashna's symptoms such as a cough, temperature, sore throat and increased mucus secretion from her cold are due to the inflammatory response and the body fighting against the virus using these defence mechanisms. The recognition of foreign proteins or compounds can have implications for medicines management. Hypersensitive reactions to medications can occur as a result of an immune response to either the drug chemical itself or a product of its metabolism. A severe immune response may result in a medical emergency known as anaphylaxis. Recognition of this and its treatment will be discussed further in Chapter 4.

As part of your understanding of normal body systems physiology, is the acknowledgement that these systems need to develop and mature, and then slowly decline as part of the natural ageing process.

The ageing process

As a nursing associate working in a variety of care settings, you will need to understand human development from conception to death. After birth, many physiological changes take place as the body matures and then begins to decline. At both ends of this age continuum, many aspects of bodily function are altered and, in some circumstances, less efficient. As well as the effects of advancing age, some of which we noted above, are concerns with developing body systems. An example is the infant's less effective temperature regulation mechanism, and this would have implications when caring for Aashna in the case study at the beginning of this chapter. Immature temperature regulation puts infants at risk of seizures associated with uncontrolled pyrexias, close observation and both pharmaceutical and non-pharmaceutical temperature-control therapies need to be advised.

Prescribing and medicines administration for infants and children require specific knowledge and skill. Pharmacokinetics and dynamics differ in children, they respond differently to medicines and doses at different stages in their development, they are therefore calculated individually according to their weight. The risk of toxicity is increased by reduced medicines clearance and differing target organ sensitivity (BNF, 2023). For those of you working with children, specific texts and guidelines are available for understanding physiology and associated safe medicines administration, and you are advised to explore these in more detail.

The process of ageing is poorly understood and affects individuals differently, and while it is not responsible for specific illnesses, it is a predisposing factor for several conditions. The lifespan of an individual is influenced by many factors including environmental and social factors, disabilities, genomics and lifestyle choices, which we will explore further in Chapter 7. Many of these factors you will have seen in your practice areas such as poverty, the effects of air pollution, and the lifestyle choices of poor diet, smoking and high alcohol intake. Increasing age is a risk factor for some disease processes, including dementia, many cancers and coronary heart disease. Increasingly, particularly in high-income countries, life expectancy has increased, and many societies and health services are needing to respond to the implications of an ageing human population. The role of preventative medicine and early interventions have become especially important. As a nursing associate, you will need to be aware of the effects that the ageing process has on physiology, the concerns this causes for prescribing medicines in all age groups, the impacts of medicines on immature systems, as well as the impacts of multiple medicines for declining body systems.

We have explored normal physiology, the effects of human development and the considerations associated with medicines management. It is now important to recognise that much of the administration of medicines is for treatment or symptom control as a result of disease processes. There are too many disease processes to discuss within this text. There are books devoted to the study of illness and associated signs and symptoms for you to increase your understanding in this area, some of which we have highlighted at the end of this chapter. To develop knowledge and understanding, you will need to explore the pathophysiology associated with disease processes for the service users in your own area of practice. You do, however, need an understanding of the general principles of disease processes, and it is to this that we shall turn to next.

Disease processes and the implications for medicines management

Pathophysiology is the study of the disordered physiological processes associated with disease or injury. It involves the understanding of **aetiology**, the defining of the cause of the disease as either genetic, congenital or acquired. Genetic cause is a mutation in a person's DNA sequence, as in Huntington's disease. Congenital causes occur when there are intrauterine problems during gestation causing abnormalities – for example, cleft palate. Acquired causality occurs when the disease is contracted after birth from others or from the environment – for example, tuberculosis (TB) or the common cold, as in Aashna's situation from the case study at the beginning of this chapter.

Signs, the objective evidence of disease, like a visible rash, and the subjective **symptoms** described, like itching, when presented, require investigation to allow for the diagnosis and prognosis – the prediction for recovery – to be made. Once diagnosed, treatment can begin to cure or, if incurable, manage the symptoms for the individual. It is this cure or symptom management that will involve, among other things, the use of medications. Recognition and understanding of the processes will allow you as nursing associates to provide high-quality, targeted care. For example, thinking about Aashna at the beginning of this chapter, we may expect a high temperature, restlessness and irritability, and increased nasal secretions as the signs of her viral cold, and advice on both pharmaceutical symptom relief like paracetamol and non-pharmaceutical alternatives like tepid bathing for temperature control should be considered. You may need to explain to Aashna's mother that antibiotics are not effective for viral infections. In addition, knowledge regarding infection control and immune responses will allow for advice regarding disease transmission and susceptibility. Thus, an understanding of both the cause (or disease process) and the pathophysiology (or effects on normal functioning and available treatment options) will allow you as a nursing associate to both explain and assist with treatment regimes.

Finally, when exploring the human body, ageing and disease processes, it is impossible to ignore the brain, our mental health and our perceptions of self and well-being. Physiology texts may simplify mental health based on two neurotransmitters, dopamine and serotonin. These chemicals allow the transmission of signals from one neuron to the next across synapses. Too little dopamine is thought to produce anxiety, while too little serotonin can lead to problems with mood control. However, recognition that we are both physical and mental entities, and that ageing and the disease processes will be influenced by both physical and psychological parameters, is important for us as healthcare professionals when caring for our service users and managing therapies, including medication. An example of this is the use of **adjuvants**, medicines that can be used for pain management because of their analgesic effect, but are primarily prescribed for other purposes. Tricyclic antidepressants, such as amitriptyline, for instance, are used to treat both pain and depression, addressing both psychological and physical symptoms. There is also growing research in the field of the gut–brain axis, exploring how these systems communicate and affect each other – for instance, the effect the stress response can have on bowel symptoms in conditions such as irritable bowel syndrome (IBS) (Ancona et al., 2021). These examples demonstrate the need to understand how the mind and body interact, and how this affects medicines management.

Understanding the theory: Pathophysiology

While the theory of altered physiology as a result of differing disease processes may seem daunting when you first consider it, it will be something you will have been observing, explaining and acting on already in your daily practice. Depending on both practice and home experiences, you will have observed the signs and symptoms of various illnesses and, with a basic understanding of how the body works, been able to explain these. You will have come across someone suffering with diarrhoea and vomiting, and seen the effects of the lack of absorption of nutrients and fluid. You will have advised rest and rehydration, and in some instances medications to relieve the physical distress, while considering the embarrassment, potential lack of dignity and psychological distress of the condition. You will also have tempered your advice and treatment options depending on the age of the individual suffering. This is an example of you putting the theory into practice.

Now that you have worked through this chapter and have explored the body and its constituents, the body systems with distinct roles in medicines management and been introduced to ageing and disease processes, take some time to reflect on what you have learnt, which will allow you to apply it to your practice. Activity 2.5 will help you with this.

Activity 2.5   Reflection

Now that you have read through the chapter, consider the following questions.

1. Describe the transport and communication systems between all the different cell types.

2. Consider why so many medications are contraindicated in hepatic and renal impairment.

3. Consider the effects of ageing on physiology and describe the implications for medicines management.

4. What does the term 'pathophysiology' mean and how does it impact on medicines management?

An outline answer is given at the end of this chapter.

Now that you have had a chance to reflect on the contents of this chapter, you can see from the following summary that you have, in fact, explored a large amount of theory and been able to link this to your own practice.

Chapter summary

As you have discovered from this chapter, our bodies function as integrated, interdependent body systems to maintain an equilibrium known as homoeostasis. In order to do this, we must take in and process nutrients through our digestive and hepatic system, metabolising and retaining those substances required and detoxifying and removing those unwanted substances, eliminating them through the liver and renal system. This chapter has outlined the body systems responsible for these processes and has discussed alterations to this function as a result of maturation and ageing. It has outlined those additional body systems essential for homoeostasis including the cardiovascular, integumentary and immune system. In addition, this chapter has defined pathophysiology as an altered physiology as a result of disease processes and has introduced the need for appropriate medicines management to manage the signs and symptoms of these processes.

The activities included in this chapter have invited you to consider the organ systems of the body, noting their main function and component organs. They have required you to consider the specific function of the digestive, hepatic and renal systems, and asked you to review these in the light of the impact on medicines management.

Activities: Brief outline answers

Activity 2.1: Critical thinking (page 24)

Within the body there are different levels of structural organisation. Cells with similar structures and functions form tissues. Organs are made up of different types of tissue and have a specific function. A number of organs and tissues that contribute to fulfil bodily function are found in body systems – for example, the digestive system. The human body has several systems that work interdependently to maintain health (see Table 2.1).

Table 2.1   The systems of the body, the organs involved and the system's main function

Organ system	Function	Tissues and organs
Cardiovascular	Continuous flow of blood with oxygen and nutrients to all cells.	Heart, blood vessels.
Respiratory	Supplies oxygen required for cell reaction to produce energy; removes carbon dioxide as waste product.	Lungs, tracheal system.
Integumentary	Protects underlying structures, contains sensory nerve endings and allows temperature regulation.	Skin. Accessory structures: glands, hair, nails.
Lymphatic	Filters and returns fluid into blood stream.	Lymph vessels and nodes, spleen, thymus, bone marrow.
Nervous	Detects and responds to changes inside and outside the body.	Brain, spinal cord, peripheral nerves.
Digestive	Alimentary canal for absorbing nutrients.	Stomach, liver, pancreas, gall bladder, bowel.
Endocrine	Secretory cells that diffuse hormones as chemical messengers to maintain homoeostasis.	Endocrine glands: pituitary, thyroid, parathyroid, adrenal cortex, pancreatic islets, pineal.
Musculoskeletal	Provides body framework and allows movement.	Bones, muscles, ligaments.
Urinary	Main excretory system.	Kidneys, ureters, urinary bladder, urethra.
Immune	Protective measures against pathogens.	Skin, lymph tissue.
Special senses	Hearing, sight, smell and taste – detects and transmits information.	Ear, eye, olfactory nerves.

Activity 2.2: Critical thinking (page 27)

1.   The endocrine glands secrete b), chemical transmitters called hormones.
2.   The smallest living unit of the human body is c), a cell.

3. The regulation of body systems to maintain equilibrium is called b), homoeostasis.

4. Fluid found inside the cell membrane is called a), intracellular.

Activity 2.3: Critical thinking (page 28)

First, the mechanical breakdown of food occurs in the mouth. This passes through the upper GI tract into the small intestine. Here, absorption occurs through the villi into the circulatory system where nutrient-rich blood is carried to the liver. The liver as the main organ of metabolism processes nutrients into useful components, as well as detoxifying harmful substances. This will include the breaking down of the meal nutrients into constituent parts and the removal by metabolism of the alcohol as a harmful, toxic substance. Contents that are not absorbed continue down the GI tract through the large intestine where water and salts are reabsorbed; this is then compacted and excreted as faeces. The kidneys meanwhile assist with filtering to ensure that essential nutrients are reabsorbed and waste products are removed through urine.

Activity 2.4: Reflection (page 29)

Inflammatory bowel disease (IBD): chronic inflammation is characterised by recurrent and prolonged tissue damage and repairing resulting in scarring. Macrophages engulf and destroy invading pathogens by phagocytosis. They kill and digest by using harmful chemicals, including digesting enzymes. These can be released into surrounding healthy tissue and damage it. Damaged tissue will be replaced by scar tissue.

- Two main forms – Crohn's disease and ulcerative colitis – a combination of causative factors; biopsy taken to definitively diagnose.
- Symptoms may include pain, bleeding and diarrhoea, altered quality of life, anaemia, weight loss, fatigue.
- Implications: reduced appetite, increased peristalsis and resultant poor nutrient absorption or constriction of passage due to scar tissue with resultant slow or absent motility. Affects ability to digest food, absorb nutrients and eliminate waste products.
- Co-morbidities: inflammation of joints, skin and eyes, liver damage.
- Symptom management with anti-inflammatories, immunosuppressants and biological therapies – for example, corticosteroids: hydrocortisone; aminosalicylates: sulfasalazine; immunosuppressants: azathioprine; biological therapies: infliximab.
- Emotional support, nutritional advice, fertility advice.

Activity 2.5: Reflection (page 34)

1. Transport systems include the cardiovascular and lymphatic system. Blood transports essential substances throughout the body, including oxygen, nutrients, chemical substances, including medications and waste products. The lymphatic system drains plasma protein, bacteria and cell debris into the bloodstream. Communication systems receive, collate and respond to information with both the internal and external environment. They include the nervous and endocrine systems.

2. Medications may be contraindicated in hepatic and renal impairment, as these are the main body systems responsible for elimination. Reduced ability to remove toxic substances due to damage, disease or ageing may prolong the effect of the medication and increase the likelihood of an adverse effect.

3. As the body matures and then begins to decline, many aspects of bodily function are altered and become less efficient. This causes concerns for the prescribing of medicines as reduced absorption, distribution metabolism and excretion will impact on dosage, frequency and types of medications prescribed. There is also the concern regarding the impacts of multiple medicines for declining body systems, known as polypharmacy.

4. Pathophysiology describes the disordered physiological processes associated with disease or injury. It forms the basis of prescribing of medications for symptom management or treatment.

Further reading

The following titles may be helpful.

Ashelford, S, Raynsford, J and Taylor, V (2024) *Pathophysiology and Pharmacology for Nursing Students*, 3rd edition. London: SAGE.

This book is a clear and readable introduction to common illnesses and the underlying pathology. This is a particularly useful resource if you want to find out more about medicines management for specific diseases.

Barber, P, Parkes, J and Blundell, D (2012) *Further Essentials of Pharmacology for Nurses*. Maidenhead: Open University Press.

This book covers specialised medicines for a range of common diseases. Pathophysiology is explored before discussing pharmacological treatment options.

Barber, P and Robertson, D (2020) *Essentials of Pharmacology for Nurses* (4th edn). Maidenhead: Open University Press.

This updated edition discusses medicines for a range of common diseases.

Brown, MJ, Sharma, P, Mir, F and Bennett, PN (2019) *Clinical Pharmacology – E-book* (12th edn). Elsevier.

This e-book discusses the key pharmacological concepts necessary for safe drug therapy in clinical practice. This is particularly useful if wanting to explore key body systems in relation to medicines management.

Herlihy, B. (2018) *The Human Body in Health and Illness* (6th edn). St Louis, MI: Elsevier.

This book covers the key concepts in relation to anatomy and physiology of the body without going into too much depth. It is easy to read and understand. It also incorporates pathophysiology within each chapter.

Minett, P and Ginesi, P (2020) *Anatomy & Physiology An introduction for nursing and healthcare*. Banbury: Lantern Publishing Ltd.

An easy and understandable book that covers the core areas of anatomy and physiology that TNA's need for practice.

Peate, I and Dryden, P (2022) *Fundamentals of Pharmacology for Children's Nurses.* Oxford: Wiley

This book focusses on pharmacological considerations for health professionals working with children and young people. It encourages person-centred care for this service user group and includes medicine optimisation, social prescribing, safety and specific considerations for babies, child and young people.

Tortora, G and Derrickson, B (2017) Tortora's *Principles of Anatomy and Physiology* (15th edn). Oxford: Wiley.

This is a comprehensive and easy-to-digest anatomy and physiology textbook commonly used by healthcare professionals.

Waugh, A and Grant, A (2018) *Ross & Wilson Anatomy and Physiology in Health and Illness* (13th edn). London: Elsevier.

This is a core text for determining body systems and how they work, supplemented by consideration of age-related changes in normal physiology and the pathophysiology of some commonly encountered disease processes.

Useful websites

The following websites are useful resources to aid your understanding.

Electronic Medicines Compendium: www.medicines.org.uk/emc

This website provides information on pharmacodynamics and kinetics

National Institute of Clinical Excellence: www.nice.org.uk

NICE guidelines are available for most conditions and diseases. It identifies aetiology, common signs and symptoms, investigations and assessments required for diagnosis and evidence-based recommendations for treatment, which include pharmacological and non-pharmacological options.

Think Kidneys: www.thinkkidneys.nhs.uk/aki/wp-content/uploads/sites/2/2016/07/Primary-Care-Advice-for-medication-review-in-AKI-.pdf

This website provides a range of resources for all healthcare professionals to raise awareness of the risks of acute kidney injury (AKI). The link provides a guide on medication that has the potential to harm the renal system.

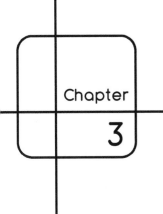

Principles of pharmacology

Chapter aims

After reading this chapter, you will be able to:

* understand the pharmacological principles for medicines management;
* appreciate the science of pharmacokinetics and pharmacodynamics, how medications affect the body and what effect the body has on the medicine itself;
* understand why certain medicines are used to prevent and treat certain conditions.

Introduction

Case study: Henry

Henry is an elderly gentleman who has learning difficulties, has type 2 diabetes and has taken medication to prevent epileptic seizures for many years. Recently, one of his medications has been changed to sodium valproate, but Henry does not remember the name of this new drug. He attends the A&E department with a painful and infected wound on his foot, having injured himself a few weeks ago. Henry informs the doctor of his previous anticonvulsant medicine, the name he is familiar with. The doctor prescribes the antibacterial ertapenem for the infection along with some painkillers. A few days later Henry has several epileptic fits.

Henry's case study is an example of the importance of understanding the basic principles of pharmacology, how medications work and possible interactions. In this fictitious scenario, Henry was unable to articulate what medications he takes and the doctor prescribed an antibiotic that reduces the plasma concentration of valproate and therefore increases the risk of therapeutic failure of the anti-convulsant medicine (BNF, 2023). In other words, the antibiotic rendered the anti-convulsant medication less effective. This raises several issues you may encounter in your practice – the need for thorough assessment and reliable communication – and underlines the necessity for examining how and why medicines work.

In Chapter 1, you were asked to consider the definition of a medicine, which was described as having properties that treat or prevent disease. In this chapter, we will examine this in more detail. We will determine the different medication forms and how this gives rise to their naming, then consider how the body acts on these chemicals via absorption, metabolism, distribution and elimination to allow safe usage and removal. Next, we will describe how these chemicals work to prevent disease or treat illnesses, and finally explore some of the factors that influence the therapeutic choice and effectiveness of medications.

In historical times, a variety of noxious substances were used as treatments. Arsenic was used for cosmetic purposes, for a paler complexion, as a stimulant and as a treatment for syphilis. In these cases, along with others, treatments were discontinued after evidence proved their harm or uselessness.

Pharmacology is the scientific study of the origin, nature, chemistry, effects and uses of medicines. These processes form the basis for why medicines are given in a particular way, why some may be given with food, why some are given more regularly than others and which medicine is the most appropriate in any given situation. This knowledge is essential to ensure accurate and safe **administration** of treatment regimens to your service users.

You may feel quite daunted when it comes to trying to remember the names of medicines and how they work, known as their mode of action, their usual dosages and possible side effects. This is a common fear among healthcare professionals, but it is neither necessary nor, in fact, possible as medications and treatment practices are constantly changing. What is important for your service users' safety is that you understand the pharmacological principles and are able to apply that knowledge within your sphere of practice. Therefore, while you do not need to memorise all drugs and their mechanisms, you do need pharmacological knowledge to look up and interpret information, and remember basic kinetics and dynamics to know how to apply the information.

Before we examine these principles in more detail, let us start with an activity to help you reflect on your current knowledge of the science of medications.

Activity 3.1   Reflection

Think of an example when you have observed, or been involved with, medicines administration at home or in a work capacity.

- What do you know about the different names given to medicines?
- What knowledge do you have about how medicines work and how they stop working within the body?
- Do you know how we group classes of medicines to describe their usage and give us some idea as to what their side effects may be?

As the answers are based on your own observation and reflection, there are no outline answers at the end of this chapter.

You may wish to discuss this reflection with colleagues and retain the information in a personal portfolio.

Having thought about your observations and prior knowledge, let us consider the science in more detail. There are three basic concepts of pharmacology. **Pharmacokinetics** explains the absorption, distribution, metabolism and excretion of medicines. This branch of pharmacology is also concerned with a drug's onset of action, peak concentration level and duration of action. **Pharmacodynamics** are the biochemical effects of the medicines, their mechanisms of action, and **pharmacotherapeutics** are the use of medicines to prevent and treat conditions. In addition, the science of pharmacology helps us to understand how medicines are derived and developed, named and classified, and chosen for administration.

Naming medicines: Nomenclature

Have you wondered why, when you are uncertain of a drug and you look it up in the *British National Formulary* (BNF), that there are several names for the same medication? This is because the medicine will have a **chemical name** describing its chemical composition and molecular structure, a **generic name**, which indicates the active ingredient of the medicine, and its **proprietary name**. This trade name is the drug title which can only be used by the patent owner, which is usually the manufacturer. So, for example, isobutylphenylpropionic acid as a chemical name indicates the non-proprietary drug ibuprofen, which is the term you should see on the prescription as it denotes the medication class. Nurofen is a proprietary trade or brand name registered by the drug manufacturer. Another example is N-acetyl-para-aminophenol, the chemical name of paracetamol, with Panadol being a brand-specific medication available to buy. This variety occurs as initially a drug company will invest large amounts of money developing a new medicine, discussed further in Chapter 7. The patent for this product usually lasts for 20 years; after this, other drug companies can produce their version of this medicine, usually a lot cheaper as they have not had the research and preclinical trial testing costs. They will use this chemical compound, and therefore generic active ingredient, but formulate their product in a slightly different way and give it a unique name.

The European Union requires manufacturers to use the **recommended International Nonproprietary Name** (rINN) for all medicines, which in many cases are identical to the British approved name. Where they had a different name, the rINN has been adopted in UK healthcare, and this is the naming you will find in the BNF. The use of the non-proprietary name on the prescription allows for the most cost-effective drug to be administered. If a brand name is used, then the brand drug must be given. Brand-specific drugs may be required if there is an established difference between a patient's response to a certain brand or if there is a requirement for slow, modified or controlled release, which may only be available in one brand.

Medicines that share similar characteristics can additionally be grouped together as a pharmacological class. Antihypertensive treatments are an example of this. To help with our understanding of the functions of these drugs, **suffixes**, or common endings, are used. Some examples include -olol for beta-blockers like propanolol and bisoprolol, -pril for angiotensin-converting enzyme inhibitors like ramipril and lisinopril. In addition, medicines can be classed or grouped dependent on their therapeutic use. So, anti-epileptics, analgesics, anti-hypertensives and anti-psychotics are all examples of therapeutic class. Now you have discovered that medications have different names and means of classification, complete Activity 3.2 in order to test your understanding.

Activity 3.2   Critical thinking

You are asked by a friend for some advice regarding an advert he has seen for a medication to relieve flu symptoms. He purchased Anadin®, which he saw advertised on television, but when he gets it home, he realises that it does not look the same as the medication he saw advertised and it does not state the same symptom relief on the box. He asks you to explain his mistake.

An outline answer is given at the end of this chapter.

Hopefully, due to your understanding of the different naming of medications and the use of brand labels, you would have been able to answer your friend's question. You may have used several sources of drug information to assist you. For example, perhaps the box label, the inserted information leaflet or you may have accessed the internet as a source of advice. As a nursing associate, you will be aware that caution is needed as the information online is not peer reviewed and accuracy cannot be assured. Finally, and most reassuringly, would be the use of the BNF as an up-to-date, comprehensive guide to medicines management, and you can access this in either book or online format. The BNF would have informed you of indications, contraindications, cautions, interactions and side effects, and it is where this information comes from that we need to explore next.

Medicines uses

Medicines may be used to prevent or treat disease, but we need to know what the indications for a specific medicine are. The **prophylactic** administration of a medicine describes the use of the drug to prevent disease, examples being a vaccine given to induce resistance, an antifibrinolytic after surgery to prevent clot formation and deep vein thrombosis or embolus or a drug given to reduce cholesterol and thus reduce the likelihood of heart disease or stroke. The **therapeutic** administration of a medicine describes the use of a drug either to treat a condition, control the disease progression or to reduce unpleasant symptoms, and you will have observed many different examples of these. Medicines may also be used to aid diagnosis – for example, fluorescein sodium is an eye drop which, although yellow in colour, when a fluorescent light is shone at it, makes lesions and foreign bodies on the cornea show up clearly with a blue glow. This, along with other eyedrops, like mydriatics that dilate the pupil, make eye examination easier. Clearly, therefore, knowing what we need the medicine to achieve aids the prescriber to choose, but it is not as simple as that. The prescriber will also need to understand in what format this medicine can be given and how it is going to work in order to predict the contraindications, cautions, interactions and side effects. We will examine these next.

Pharmacokinetics: What the body does to the medicine

Derived from the Greek words *pharmakon*, meaning drug, and *kinetics*, meaning motion, pharmacokinetics describes what the body does to a medication. In other words, once administered through any route, which is explored in Chapter 4, it describes the effect the various bodily functions have on the chemical. It explores how the body allows and influences the absorption, how the chemical is distributed around the body, how it is broken down, known as metabolism, and how it is removed from the body or excreted. We will examine each of these in turn.

Absorption in pharmacology is the movement of a drug from the site of administration to the bloodstream. Since medicines can be given through a variety of routes, this will have the initial effect on how the medicinal chemical is absorbed. Most medicines in common use are swallowed and are therefore absorbed by passing from the stomach into the intestines, passing through the liver, and from there into the bloodstream, or circulatory system (see Chapter 2). Medicines given by other routes enter the blood directly from the site of administration. Intramuscularly and subcutaneously, through the capillary blood supply of the muscle and skin, and topically through the mucosal membrane at the site where the medication is deposited – for example, the rectum, vagina and nasal passages. Medicines administered by inhalation are atomised into droplets and nebulised medicines are aerosolised. They are then absorbed into the pulmonary circulatory system.

In order to pass into the circulatory system, the medicinal chemical needs to pass across cell membranes and it does this by passive diffusion, facilitated diffusion or active transport. **Passive diffusion**, as the name suggests, occurs passively without the requirement for any energy or effort. One side of the cell membrane will have a greater concentration of the substance and the molecules will move along the **concentration gradient** to the area where there is a lesser concentration, as a way of evening out the substance on both sides. The word 'diffusion' derives from the Latin word to spread out.

Facilitated diffusion, as the name suggests, requires something to facilitate or allow this process to happen. Carrier proteins are required to move the substance, in this case the medicinal chemical, across the cell membrane from the area of high to low concentration, and they do this by binding to the drug chemical.

Active transport requires energy. Our body's energy is in the form of adenosine triphosphate (ATP) to move the medicine molecules across the cell membrane, because they are either being moved against a concentration gradient or because the molecules are so large (Figure 3.1).

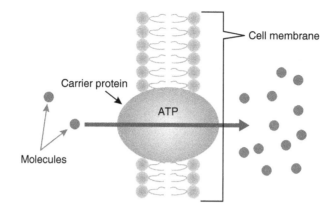

Figure 3.1 Passive and facilitated diffusion and active transport

Source: Cook et al. (2021).

Most medicines are absorbed by diffusion through the wall of the intestine into the circulatory system, and this process will occur more quickly if the medicine molecules are small and lipid-soluble, drugs are usually manufactured to make them as lipid-soluble as possible. It is also worth noting here that non-ionised molecules are more lipid-soluble than ionised molecules. Any molecule, medicines included, consists of two or more **atoms**. Atoms are electrically neutral, consisting of a balance of positively charged **protons** and negatively charged **electrons**. When they lose or gain an electrical charge, they become **ions** and thus we describe these as ionised. Some medicines are deliberately formulated or manufactured as less lipid-soluble, however, to allow them to reach the colon largely unabsorbed – for example, aminosalicylates which are used in the treatment of ulcerative colitis.

Fewer drugs are absorbed by active transport and some examples include levodopa, iron and fluorouracil, as well as electrolytes, such as sodium and potassium. A unique form of active transport called **pinocytosis** occurs when a cell engulfs a drug molecule; the fat-soluble vitamins, A, D, E and K, are absorbed in this manner.

Absorption rate describes the time from when the medicine is administered to its entry into the bloodstream and thus will be affected by several factors. The fewer cells separating the medicine from the bloodstream and the larger the surface area, the quicker the absorption; sublingual and inhalatory medications are absorbed quickly. The more complex membrane system of the gut mucosa, muscles and skin result in slower medicine absorption. In addition, medicines absorbed from the gastrointestinal tract will enter the **portal** circulation, which will transport the drug directly to the liver, where some are extensively broken down as they pass through, known as **first-pass metabolism**. In other words, the liver metabolises much of the drug before it reaches the general or systemic circulation. This means that only a proportion of the medicine absorbed will reach the general circulation and be carried to the site of action, known as the **bioavailability**. Glyceryl trinitrate (GTN) as an example shows a very significant first-pass effect, and as such is given sublingually for the treatment of angina. Other medicines that show significant first-pass effect may still be given orally, but the dosage will need to reflect this in order to ensure a therapeutic effect. The greater the blood flow to the absorption site, the quicker absorption may happen, and thus the onset of the medicinal action. Hot and cold environments, the general health of the individual and choice of administration site will have an impact. Pain, stress, malnutrition, general malaise and stomach contents may also slow medication absorption, as will the individual's characteristics. These characteristics, such as their age and ethnicity will be explored in more detail later. The formulation, or type of the medicine, will additionally have an impact. Liquid medicines are readily absorbed, whereas enteric-coated drugs are specifically formulated so that they do not dissolve immediately in the stomach, but rather release the active ingredient in the small intestine.

Distribution, as the name suggests, is how the medicine is distributed around the body where it must then penetrate the body tissues to cause an effect, as relatively few medicines exert their pharmacological action in the blood itself. Most medicines therefore need to move from the blood into the interstitial fluid, which surrounds the cell, to interact with the cell membrane target proteins, examined further when we discover how medicines act on the body. As with absorption, distribution is affected by blood flow or tissue perfusion; those organs with a large blood supply, including the heart, liver and kidneys, will receive the medicinal product quicker than other internal organs. The size, solubility, polarity and the acidity of the medicine in solution will additionally affect its distribution. Lipid-soluble drugs easily cross cell membranes, whereas water-soluble medicines cannot. Finally, the affinity or how avidly a drug can bind to plasma proteins will affect distribution. Many medicinal molecules do not dissolve in the blood, but are bound to plasma proteins such as albumin. The drug binds to these proteins, but it is only the unbound chemical that will have a medicinal effect. Thus, it is important to remember conditions that reduce the amount of plasma protein or albumin, like malnutrition or severe burns, will leave more of the free unbound medicine in the bloodstream able to exert a medicinal effect. This may result in a greater response to the medication and additionally greater susceptibility to unwanted effects. Some medicines have a higher affinity for plasma proteins and as such may take longer to move from the blood to the target cell. Warfarin is an example: it has a long **half-life**. This is the time it takes for the plasma concentration of the medicine to fall by half of its original value. This therefore causes a prolonged anticoagulant effect, taking many days for its pharmacological effects to stop after the administration has been stopped. In addition, some medicines will have an affinity for the same plasma protein. Warfarin and aspirin are good examples, competing to bind to the same protein. If administered together, aspirin will bind to the plasma protein, displacing the warfarin and as such making the free warfarin able to exert its anticoagulant effect to a greater degree.

Distribution will also be affected if there are barriers that medicines cannot penetrate. One such example is the membrane barrier that separates the circulating blood and the cerebral spinal fluid. Known as the **blood–brain barrier**, this membrane, which is designed to protect the brain from harmful substances such as bacteria, also prevents the movement of all but the very small medicinal molecules. This can make administering medicines to have a therapeutic effect on the brain difficult. Some molecules do pass this barrier easily, however – for example, alcohol and diazepam. There are also variations in the ability for medicines to pass across the **placenta** from mother to unborn child. Lipid-soluble drugs will cross much easier than water-soluble ones, but once the medication has crossed, its elimination is slow. Medicines may also be from mother to infant through breast milk. Antidepressants as an example, pre and postnatally, require careful prescribing weighting up risks and benefits for mother and baby. In addition, prescribers will need to be aware that physiological changes that occur during pregnancy will have implications for medicine distribution. The concentration of albumin, one of the plasma proteins, is reduced due to the increase in circulatory volume during pregnancy, which will increase the amount of free and active medicine molecules in the blood.

Metabolism is the term used to describe the body's ability to change the medicine molecule from its dosage form to a more water-soluble form to allow it to be removed from the body. This metabolism is also known as **biotransformation**, where the medicine is converted or transformed into inactive components or metabolites. However, some medicines are formulated so that they are inactive until they are altered or metabolised by the body, known as prodrugs. In this way, they only become active and cause a medicinal effect once they are metabolised or biotransformed. An example of this is valaciclovir, the prodrug for aciclovir.

Most medicines are metabolised by enzymes in the liver, although metabolism may also occur in the plasma, kidneys and intestinal membranes. Those metabolised in the wall of the gut have a clinical significance if food substances such as grapefruit juice, which can inhibit gut enzyme function, are present. Other factors will affect the body's ability to metabolise medicines. If the same enzymes are required – for example, to break down two or more medicines – then this competition will allow for the accumulation of one of the drugs, increasing the potential for toxicity or an adverse reaction. Some disease processes will affect metabolism, including cirrhosis of the liver and heart failure, which may reduce the circulation to the liver. Genetics and a person's age may play a part. Some people are better able to metabolise drugs, and developmental changes, including small, under-developed livers in infants and declining liver size and function in old age, will affect biotransformation. Additionally, some environmental factors such as stress, anxiety or smoking can slow medicine metabolism.

Excretion refers to the elimination of the medicine from the body. Most medicines are excreted by the kidneys and the inactive components or metabolites leave the body in the urine. Thus, it is important to consider the impact of kidney disease on this process. Care is required for medicines management for those with kidney impairment. Drugs may also be excreted through the lungs, in expired breaths, through exocrine glands, through the intestinal tract into the faeces and through the skin, secreted in sweat. Amiodarone, rifampicin and vecuronium – medicines with large molecular weight – are examples of drugs eliminated by the liver in bile and excreted in faeces.

For manufacturers and those prescribing, it is important to understand how long a medicine remains in the body and able to exert an effect, so that it is possible to determine how often a medicine needs to be taken. To aid with this, the half-life of the drug is determined, identifying how long it takes for half of the administered drug to be eliminated. This time will be affected by the rates of absorption, distribution, metabolism and excretion. In addition, three other factors determine how long a medicine can exert an effect; the **onset of action** refers to the time taken for the medicine to start working once it has been administered. **Peak concentration** describes the point when the absorption rate equals the elimination rate and thus there is a peak amount of the drug available. **Duration of action** is the time the medicine continues to produce its therapeutic, diagnostic or preventative effect.

So, having explored and understood what the body will do to our medicine, and therefore what format and how often we may need to deliver our chemical to allow it to have an effect, we need to consider how these medicine molecules produce the effects they do.

Pharmacodynamics: What the medicine does to the body

Pharmacodynamics is the study of the various mechanisms that produce the physiological or biochemical effect. It is the study of the body's reactions to the medicinal molecules.

Medicine as a replacement: in certain cases, the medicine will bring about a normal physiological response as a replacement or substitute for a deficiency – for example, synthetic insulins for service users with diabetes mellitus, ferrous sulphate for iron-deficiency anaemias and levothyroxine for service users with under-active thyroids.

Most medicines, however, produce their biochemical effect in cells and do this by targeting key cell membrane proteins, which can be divided into four categories: receptors, enzymes, ion channels and carrier proteins.

Receptors: receptor proteins on the cell membrane usually respond to the body's natural chemicals, transmitter substances, mediators or hormones. The medicines therefore can mimic the body's natural chemical and activate the receptor, these are called **agonists**. It does this as the medicine's molecular structure is similar in shape to the body's natural chemical – think of it as a specific key to open a specific lock. Alternatively, the medicine can combine with the receptor and not activate it; these are known as **antagonists**. This time the key fits but does not open the lock. These antagonists may either bind with the receptor and block it so that the body's normal chemicals cannot activate it or simply reduce the function of the receptor. Naloxone is an example of an opioid antagonist. The **affinity** the medicine has for the receptor describes the strength of the bond between the two. In addition, the ability the medicine has to bind or combine with one particular type of receptor describes its **specificity**. In other words, the medicine is quite selective to one receptor. No medicines are truly specific, however, and thus can not only produce a therapeutic effect but also can produce additional unwanted effects, known as side effects. The relationship between a medicine's desired effect and the adverse effects is called the **therapeutic index**, also known as the **margin of safety**. In other words, a medicine may have a very narrow range of safety between an effective dose and a lethal one (Figure 3.2).

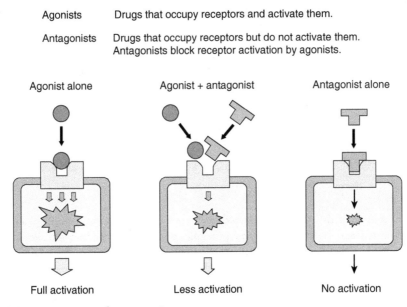

Agonists	Drugs that occupy receptors and activate them.
Antagonists	Drugs that occupy receptors but do not activate them. Antagonists block receptor activation by agonists.

Agonist alone   Agonist + antagonist   Antagonist alone

Full activation   Less activation   No activation

Figure 3.2 Agonists and antagonists

Source: Ashelford et al. (2024)

Enzyme inhibitors: medicines may interact with the body's enzymes which are responsible for promoting or accelerating normal biochemical reactions. Within each cell there are thousands of tiny biochemical reactions that require enzymes as catalysts or required substance to allow the reaction to happen. Medicines are formulated to inhibit or prevent them from performing their role. This inhibition is caused by the medicine binding to the active site of the enzyme where it would usually allow the conversion of one substance into another by being formulated to have a similar molecular shape – the key blocking the lock again. Ibuprofen, a non-steroidal anti-inflammatory (NSAID), is an example of a cyclooxygenase (COX) enzyme inhibitor. The enzyme cyclooxygenase is required to facilitate the production of prostaglandins, chemicals that promote inflammation, pain and fever. NSAIDs work by reducing the production of prostaglandins and thus reducing these symptoms. Further examples include the monoamine oxidase inhibitors, which are anti-depressants, carbonic anhydrase inhibitors, which are diuretics, and statins such as pravastatin and atorvastatin which block the enzyme pathway that produces cholesterol in the liver.

Affecting transport processes: these medicines, as the name suggests, act on the movement of molecules. **Ion channels** are selective pores in the membrane of the cell which allow the transfer of ions. Think of them like tunnels with barriers that allow atoms which have lost or gained an electrical charge to pass along. These pores, or barriers, are opened or closed either by electrical means with the charged potential of the membrane or by chemical transmitter substances. Thus, medicines formulated to act on these channels do so either by inserting themselves in the channel, blocking it and preventing ion movement, or by modulating or changing how the ion channel behaves, enhancing or inhibiting their action. Some examples of these medicines that will act on these pores or openings are calcium-channel blockers, widely used in the treatment of angina; local anaesthetics which block the sodium channels in nerves; anxiolytics which reduce anxiety, like diazepam; antihypertensives like verapamil and some anticonvulsants.

Carrier proteins additionally affect the movement of molecules and are divided into two main categories. In the first group, some proteins will transport ions across the cell membrane using ATP as the energy source in the form of ion pumps, which can be found in various parts of the body. Frusemide is an example of a diuretic that inhibits an ion carrier in the loop of Henle in the kidney, causing an increase in urine production. The second group of carrier proteins are neurotransmitter transporters affecting the junctions between neurons. Fluoxetine and paroxetine, as anti-depressants, are examples of medicines that block the carrier proteins for the neurotransmitter serotonin, although why increased synaptic serotonin levels reduce depressive symptoms is not well understood.

Understanding the theory: Pharmacokinetics and pharmacodynamics

At the beginning of this chapter we stated that it is important for your service users' safety that you understand the pharmacological principles of medicines and that you should be able to apply that knowledge within your sphere of practice. It may seem like there has been a lot of theory here for you to read and understand. We know that this theory can seem complex and daunting; however, let us think of how you are already putting this theory into practice. Think of an occasion when you have taken, or observed someone else take, a mild painkiller to relieve a lower back pain or other soft tissue injury. You will be aware of how quickly the symptoms went away, the painkiller's onset of action and then when the pain started to reoccur, the duration of action, when there was a need to take a further dose to be comfortable again as the rate of elimination was higher than the absorption rate and the peak concentration had lowered. Now think of a time when you or a friend may have taken a strong painkiller, or maybe consumed a little too much alcohol, and the effect it had. Did one of you seem to suffer the sedation effects quicker because you had not eaten, the rate of absorption being quicker due to an empty stomach? Was one of you more affected because of age, ethnicity, sex or a health condition – all of the things that can affect distribution and metabolism? Later that day, did you have to increase your trips to the toilet as your body attempted to eliminate the foreign chemical in your urine – in this case, alcohol or painkiller? Finally, were you concerned about driving home or even driving the next day due to an awareness of how long the alcohol, or analgesic with its sedative effect, was in your system waiting to be completely eliminated? An awareness of how substances, like commonly taken medications or dietary molecules such as alcohol, affect us all will help to put the theory into practice.

Factors influencing medicinal effects

In discussing the pharmacokinetics and dynamics of medicines, we have begun to explore some of the factors that will influence the choice of medication for a service user. We have discovered what happens to the medicine when it enters the body and what effects the medicine exerts. No two people are the same, however, and most drug trials are usually undertaken with healthy, young individuals. The clinical setting and therapeutic use may vary considerably. As a nursing associate, part of the healthcare team responsible for medicines management, you will want to consider several factors before administering any medicine and we will give some thought to those now.

Weight: the recommended dose of a medicine is usually based on evaluation studies from an 'average' weight individual, usually estimated to be around 70 kg. Thus, your service users who are much heavier or indeed lighter than this 'average' person may require adjusted doses to achieve the required therapeutic response or avoid toxic effects.

Gender: physiological differences exist between the sexes. Women have more adipose, or fat cells, than men and so medicines deposited in fat may be released slower and have a prolonged duration of action. For example, inhalation anaesthetics given for surgery have an affinity for depositing in fat and thus may have a prolonged sedative effect in female patients.

Genetics can explain varying responses to medicines, usually related to underactive or overactive enzyme metabolism. It is difficult to predict how an individual from any race may react to a medicine, but **pharmacogenomics** – the study that explores unique differences to medicines based on genetic make-up –to predict this with more certainty. Currently in the UK we have one class of medication with ethnically derived guidelines. The ACE (angiotension-converting-enzyme) inhibitors – captopril, enalapril and ramipril – are not recommended as first-line antihypertensive therapy for those from an Afro-Caribbean origin due to their naturally lower circulating renin levels. ACE inhibitors act on the renin–angiotensin system. Precision medicine, where medications are tailored to individual's genetic make-up is a growing phenomenon with exciting prospects for future treatment regimens, particularly in the field of oncology.

Age: service users at the two ends of the age continuum present concerns for medicines management. Infants and children metabolise medicines differently from adults, due to immature body systems. The rate at which they metabolise and eliminate medicines may be slower for some medicines, but faster than adults for others. It is not possible to generalise and while dosage is often calculated based on the child's weight, the safest option is to prescribe and administer as few medicines as possible to children. Specialist publications like the *BNF for Children* will assist you in caring for these service users. Older adults conversely may undergo physical changes associated with the ageing process (see Chapter 2), with the resultant effect on the pharmacokinetics of medicines. However, it is not possible to generalise. The variations in lived experience, health conditions and the ageing process will make this group particularly challenging for medicines management. Declining liver and kidney function will affect the pharmacokinetics, as will the prescribing of multiple medicines for a variety of conditions. A decline in the function of one body system may result in the decline of another and so on, resulting in the need for a variety of medicines to maintain homoeostasis.

Polypharmacy is the term given to the prescribing of more than four different medicines to one individual (RPS, 2023) and it is a challenge in the older population. The potential for interactions increases with the number of medicines being taken. Further concerns include the potential for side effects to be mistaken for the normal ageing processes, and the co-morbidities of poor eyesight, cognitive function and physical abilities affecting the ability to adhere to treatment regimens.

Psychological attitudes to treatments will influence the effectiveness of a medicine. Known as the **placebo effect**, an individual's belief in the value of the medicine has been shown to affect how the drug works. A positive belief in the medicine has been shown to increase the likelihood not only of the success of the treatment regimen but also of the individual's commitment to the process. As a nursing associate, you can influence this positivity by ensuring that service users have all the information they require regarding their medication.

Tolerance: some service users may become tolerant to a medicine over time. This may occur due to increased rate of metabolism, increased resistance to the effects or other pharmacokinetic factors. As the medicine no longer produces the desired effect, a review of the therapy is required. As a nursing associate, you will be well placed to observe and respond to such situations and relay information to the prescriber. An example of medication tolerance occurs with the opioid analgesics. Service users may find previous satisfaction with a dose of painkiller is no longer true. The longer morphine as an opioid is taken, the more tolerant the body becomes to it and the analgesic effect decreases. This becomes a challenge in clinical practice for those service users with chronic pain conditions with prescribed regimens, in addition to those service users who may have taken this class of medication illicitly.

Accumulation can occur if the service user takes successive doses of a medicine more frequently than advised. This may be due to cognitive impairment, causing a lack of understanding, or forgetting that medicines have already been taken, or a lack of compliance as it may be easier to take all medicines at once. Accumulation may also occur if the body is unable to eliminate or excrete the medicine adequately. Again, in these situations as a nursing associate you will be well placed to intervene.

Environment can affect the success of medicine therapy. As discussed earlier, temperature may affect the circulatory system of your service user and consequently affect tissue perfusion, and medicine absorption and distribution. In addition, environmental factors like the products of smoking in the air and stressful situations can affect medicine metabolism.

Immunological: service users can develop an allergy to a medicine; after exposure to the chemical, a person may develop antibodies as part of the body's natural defence against the unknown. This can result in a sensitivity to the medicine with resultant unpleasant symptoms or a life-threatening anaphylaxis, discussed in more detail in Chapter 4.

Pathology/medical conditions: disease can change the chemical reactions within the body, as well as affect the pharmacokinetics. Disease processes may influence tissue perfusion, reduce circulatory flow, affect renal function, reduce metabolism due to liver disease or speed up metabolism due to infection. In addition, the presence of disease and symptom management increases the chances of polypharmacy and interactions, as well as symptoms such as diarrhoea, vomiting and pain, affecting absorption and distribution of medicines.

Nutritional status, including anorexia, obesity and poor lifestyle choices can affect how a medicine is absorbed. Service users with greater fat deposits may suffer the prolonged duration of the action of medicines which are deposited in lipids. Service users with less body mass will have less muscle and fat mass, and fewer circulating plasma proteins necessary for the pharmacokinetics and dynamics of medicines management.

Now that you have read this chapter and have explored the pharmacological principles associated with medicines management, take some time to reflect on what you have learnt, which will allow you to apply it to your practice. Activity 3.3 will help you with this.

Activity 3.3   Critical thinking

Reviewing the case study at the beginning of this chapter, consider Henry's situation. Complete the following activity to demonstrate your understanding of the pharmacological considerations discussed in this chapter.

> Henry is an elderly gentleman who has learning difficulties, is diabetic and has taken medication to prevent epileptic seizures for many years. Recently, one of his medications has been changed to sodium valproate, but Henry does not remember the name of this new drug. He attends the A&E department with a painful and infected wound on his foot, having injured himself a few weeks ago. Henry informs the doctor of his previous anticonvulsant medicine, the name he is familiar with. The doctor prescribes the antibacterial ertapenem for the infection along with some painkillers. A few days later, Henry has several epileptic fits.

Henry took his Epilim®, his anti-convulsant medication, after his breakfast in the morning prior to attending A&E. He knows he needs to take his next dose after his evening meal. The A&E team assessed Henry's condition, including an exploration of what they believed was his current medication and then administered the antibiotic ertapenem into a venous cannula once that day for the infection.

- Why are there three different names or descriptions within this chapter for Henry's medicine?
- What are the pharmacokinetic effects to be considered in this case?
- What are the pharmacodynamic effects to be considered in this case?
- What are the person-centred care issues to be considered in this case?

An outline answer is given at the end of this chapter.

You have now had the chance to reflect on the contents of this chapter and, as you can see from the summary below, that you have, in fact, explored a large amount of theory and been able to link this to your own practice.

Chapter summary

This chapter has covered the basic principles of pharmacology. You should now understand not only how medicines affect the body, known as the pharmacodynamics, but what effect the body has on the medicine, known as the pharmacokinetics. You have explored factors that may affect these processes, which will allow you to safely administer medicines to your service users. This knowledge will help you to understand the therapeutic usages of groups of medicines and to predict the side effects. Through undertaking the activities, you have been able to demonstrate your understanding and show how you can put the theory into practice. Any areas you were not sure about you can develop by rereading the appropriate section in the book or by seeking out further explanation from the suggested further reading and websites included below.

Activities: Brief outline answers

Activity 3.2: Critical thinking (page 42)

Anadin® is a brand or trade name and not a specific chemical formula or class of medication. Anadin® for symptom relief can be bought as Anadin® extra, which contains aspirin, paracetamol and caffeine, as Anadin® original, which contains aspirin and caffeine, or as Anadin® paracetamol, which just contains the chemical N-acetyl-para-aminophenol. Due to the medications contained within, they will provide different therapeutic responses and potential side effects.

Activity 3.3: Critical thinking (page 50)

Henry's medication Epilim® is the brand name, sodium valproate the recommended international non-proprietary name and anti-convulsant the therapeutic class of the drug. The fact that Henry took his sodium valproate after his breakfast in the morning tells us that this oral medicine can be absorbed through the gut mucosa and that it has a moderate onset of action, the time taken for the medicine to start working. It has a moderate duration of action time, as it only needs to be taken twice a day. That the medication is taken after food suggests that this will slow down the absorption rate, as potentially will the pain, stress and general malaise that Henry may be suffering due to the wound in his foot. The antibiotic ertapenem was given intravenously, so administered directly into the circulatory system for the quickest distribution to the site required; thus, it has not been subject to first-pass metabolism as it has not entered the general circulation via the portal system. We do not know Henry's weight, genetic make-up, age or whether he has a positive attitude to his medicine, but we do know that this may influence the effectiveness of this drug. We also know that Henry has another medical condition, diabetes, and this may affect his nutritional status, and that he is elderly, both of which can influence the effect of medication. On assessment, the A&E team did not indicate that he had either a tolerance, accumulation or immunological response to the medication as this would have caused them to review the treatment regimen. We know that Henry had a cognitive impairment which led him to fail to remember that his medication had been changed recently, which ultimately led to the pharmacodynamic effects, the reduction in plasma concentration of the valproate responsible for the adverse reaction he suffered a few days later and the return of his seizures.

Further reading

To better understand the pharmacological principles for medicines management and the science of pharmacokinetics and pharmacodynamics, as well as why certain medicines are used to prevent and treat certain conditions, the following titles may be helpful.

Ashelford, S, Raynsford, J and Taylor, V (2024) *Pathophysiology and Pharmacology for Nursing Students* (3rd edn). London: SAGE.

Barber, P and Robertson, D (2020) *Essentials of Pharmacology for Nurses* (4th edn). Maidenhead: Open University Press.

McFadden, R (2019) *Introducing Pharmacology for Nursing and Healthcare* (3rd edn). Abingdon: Routledge.

Neal, MJ (2020) *Medical Pharmacology at a Glance* (9th edn). Chichester: Wiley Blackwell.

Spires, A and O'Brien, M. (2011) *Introduction to Medicines Management in Nursing.* Exeter: Learning Matters.

Useful websites

The following websites are useful resources to aid your understanding.

British National Formulary: www.bnf.org

This website allows you to search for specific pharmacological information.

EMC: www.medicines.org.uk

This website provides up-to-date, approved and regulated prescribing and patient information for licensed medicines.

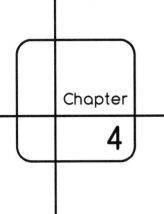

Chapter 4

Safe medicines administration

(Continued)

Part 2: Procedures for provision of person-centred nursing care

10.4   administer medication via oral, topical and inhalation routes.
10.5   administer injections using subcutaneous and intramuscular routes and manage injection equipment.
10.6   administer and monitor medications using enteral equipment.
10.7   administer enemas and suppositories.
10.8   manage and monitor effectiveness of symptom relief medication.
10.9   undertake safe storage, transportation and disposal of medicinal products.
10.10   recognise and respond to adverse or abnormal reactions to medications, and when and how to escalate any concerns.

Chapter aims

After reading this chapter, you will be able to:

•   understand the principles of safe and effective administration and optimisation of medicines in accordance with local and national policies;
•   demonstrate the ability to recognise the effects of medicines, allergies, drug sensitivity, side effects, contraindications and adverse reactions.

Introduction

Case study: George

You are a trainee nursing associate on a practice learning opportunity in the community. You visit George in his own home to participate in the prescribed dressing of this client's ulcerated legs and to assist him with taking his medication. George is known to have a heart condition requiring him to take digoxin tablets and a wound infection for which he is taking a course of antibiotics, in a syrup form. On checking George's vital signs, he is supported to take his antibiotics but not his digoxin as his pulse is only 50. While the district nurse is out of the room washing her hands, George confides that he has been having a lot of pain in his legs recently and has found taking his wife's oramorph at night has helped him get off to sleep and has been a great relief. You are concerned that the oramorph medication has not been prescribed for George and that his pain is not being appropriately managed.

George's case study is an example of the importance of safe medicines administration and raises several issues you may encounter in your practice. Throughout this chapter, we will refer to George's case study and discuss the concerns identified within it.

In the first chapter of this book, you were introduced to the legal, regulatory and governance requirements for medicines administration. We now need to explore the ethical considerations for the administration of medicines as well as the procedural skills associated with safe practice (NMC, 2018a). This chapter will help you understand and feel confident in doing this by first describing the ethical principles of consent and associated concordance, and the principles of capacity and covert medicines administration. Next, this chapter will describe the procedural skills to ensure your safe administration by highlighting the 'rights' of medicines management, describing the different routes of medicines administration and the associated administration procedures. Finally, this chapter will explore what can go wrong with medicines administration and explain adverse drug reactions (ADRs) and anaphylaxis, and your role in managing, escalating and documenting these.

While it will be for your employing organisation to determine the extent of the nursing associate role for medicines administration within your practice area (HEE, 2017), demonstration of your safety and proficiency will be required to achieve qualification, join and remain on the register (NMC, 2018a).

Patients' rights: Ethical considerations

As you discovered when reading George's case study at the beginning of this chapter, increasingly patients are being encouraged to take responsibility for their own medicines management. They need to be included more in the decision-making when selecting therapies and courses of treatment, re-enabling them to self-care. The term 'medicines optimisation' is used to underline the requirement for person-centred care, to obtain the maximum benefit for individual patients with the minimum of risk (RPS, 2023). This philosophy encourages patients to be partners in the choice of medicines and therapies, and in doing so improve patient compliance and adherence to treatments.

One of the fundamental ways to ensure your service users' understanding and participation in medicines management is to discuss all aspects of this process as part of their consent to treatment.

Consent, put simply, is the right of any adult human being of sound mind to determine what should be done with their own body. Without such consent, a healthcare profession may be deemed to have committed assault, for which they may be liable for damages. It is essential that consent is gained for all medicines administration. If you are administering an injection and a patient offers their arm and rolls up their sleeve, you are entitled to believe they are consenting for you to proceed; inferred by their actions, this is known as **implied** consent. You may assume, when administering any medication, that consent to treatment has been sought by the prescriber, and that the service user has a clear appreciation and understanding of the facts, known as **informed consent**. However, being an accountable professional, you will need to check the validity of this consent. You will need to be certain that the service user has a knowledge of the benefits of the treatment, knows any risks, and that all questions have been answered fully and honestly. The NMC state that it is deceptive to administer medicines without informed consent.

This full and honest disclosure when gaining consent may additionally need to include discussing discontinuation of treatment when the benefits are no longer present, and this can be a challenging task. You may need to discuss discontinuation of aggressive treatments and instigation of palliative medicines for patients with terminal conditions, or a discontinuation of treatment for service users with mental health conditions where they are no longer able to maintain function. In the mental health field, the concept of recovery has many definitions, but traditionally it is taken to reflect when a service user can retake control and responsibility over their lives. The stated aim of the medicines management is supporting the service user's self-efficacy in managing the pharmacological treatment. They may wish to titrate their medications against their subjective experience of illness or wellness, as psychotropic medications will have an individual response. As each person will react differently to the same dose of a medicine, there is an ethical and clinical requirement to engage the service user in the treatment regime to allow a mutual assessment of the effects on mental and physical health.

Patients have the right to refuse medication that they have previously discussed and agreed to, and withdraw their consent. As a nursing associate, you need to respect their wishes if they are deemed to have capacity. **Capacity** is defined as the state of being able to make a specific decision, at a specific time, and relies on five key principles. The Mental Capacity Act 2005; HMSO, 2005 protects those individuals who cannot make decisions for themselves and states that a person lacks capacity if they are unable to make a specific decision, at a specific time, because of an impairment of, or disturbance, in the functioning of the brain. To adhere to its principles, you must assume that a person has capacity unless proven otherwise. You cannot treat people as incapable of deciding unless all practicable steps have been tried to help them. A person should not be treated as incapable of deciding just because their decision is thought to be unwise. You must always make decisions for individuals without capacity in their best interest and finally, before deciding, you need to consider whether the outcome could be achieved in a less restrictive way. There are several implications for healthcare professionals. These include involving the patient and their significant others to ascertain what is in the individual's best interests, being aware that capacity can change over time, that individuals may have a declared **advocate** or a **lasting power of attorney (LPA)** to make decisions for them and, if necessary, care decisions may need to be referred to the court of protection for a ruling. In addition, you may be involved in caring for individuals who have been deprived of their liberty, protected currently with **deprivation of liberty safeguards (DOLS)** and when implemented the Mental Capacity (Amendment) Act 2019 (HMSO, 2019) will protect with **liberty protection safeguards** the Mental Capacity (Amendment) Act 2019 (HMSO, 2019).

This gaining of patients' trust and ensuring their understanding of medicines regimens ensures **concordance** or agreement. This concordance demonstrates a partnership of shared decision-making where a negotiated agreement exists as to whether, when and how medicines are to be taken, and embodies the notion of an alliance and the essence of informed consent. There are complexities to consider when caring for children and adults with cognitive impairment. Non-adherence to medicines regimens by service users is a common problem, in all fields of medicine, and can be covert, intentional or unintentional. This can have serious consequences for both the service user and healthcare resources.

In addition to the rights of adults with capacity to determine treatments, it is now enshrined in United Kingdom law that minors can also give consent, without the need for parental permission or knowledge. Since the legal case of Gillick versus West Norfolk and Wisbech Area Health Authority (1985), it has been clear that a minor under the age of 16 can give consent if he or she understands the consequences of their actions. Those responsible for the treatment of service users under the age of 16 will make judgements based on a clear competency assessment, sometimes referred to as **Gillick competence** to determine the child's capacity to understand fully what is proposed. **Fraser guidelines** assist healthcare providers to provide contraception and sexual health advice and treatment to minors. It is always best practice in service areas caring for minors to communicate all treatment options to both children and their parents or guardians, if you are able, to gain cooperation, consent and concordance to treatment regimes.

Covert administration is the term given when medication is administered to individuals who are unable to give informed consent to treatment and who refuse tablets or liquid preparations when they are openly offered. Covertly, healthcare professionals and carers may hide medications in food and drink, therefore disguising its presence. You must be able to make the distinction between those who refuse and are aware of the reasons for that refusal and therefore respect their decision, and those who lack capacity to make a rational decision (RPS, 2023). In addition, you need to recognise those patients who do not need their medications disguising, as they are unaware they are receiving it, and those to whom deception is necessary.

As outlined in Chapter 1, the Mental Capacity Act 2005; 2019 Amendment Bill (HMSO, 2005, 2019) provides a statutory framework to empower and protect vulnerable people who may not be able to make their own decisions. It makes clear who can make decisions and in which circumstances. If a person is lawfully detained under a section of the Mental Health Act 2007; HMSO, 2007, some forms of forced or disguised medications are recognised by law. A decision may be made either to save a patient's life, reduce suffering, prevent a condition from worsening or to prevent certain behaviour being a danger to the patient or others. In these circumstances, you will need to refer to the Act, codes of practice and employers' policies. These treatments can be administered in the short term before independent second opinions must be sought and clear procedures followed. In these circumstances, you will need to work within your employing organisation's covert administration of medicines policies and procedures, and you need to be aware of the aims, intent and implications of such practice to ensure professional accountability. The decision to give covert medication is a multidisciplinary team decision and NICE (2019a), PrescQUIPP (2022) and CQC (2022b) have all produced guidance on issues to be considered, while recommending that covert administration should be a last resort.

Understanding the theory: Ethical considerations

While the theory of consent, capacity and concordance may seem intimidating when you first consider it, it can be quite simple and something you have been doing already in your daily practice. Any time you have cared for a service user and explained what you are doing and why, discussing their care choices and assessed how well they understand what is going on, you have been ensuring their right to choose, promoting compliance with their care and ensuring your own personal integrity. This is an example of you putting the theory into practice.

Once consent is established and treatment regimens have been agreed, then the principles of safe and effective administration and optimisation of medicines requires several steps to ensure safe medicines administration.

'Rights' of medicines administration

There are several steps that you should use to minimise the potential for an error when assisting your patients with taking their medications. These are commonly referred to as the 'rights' of medicines administration and, depending on the sources read, these can be a variety of numbered steps. We are suggesting eight 'rights' of administration, which suggest that you check you have the right patient, the right medication for them, the right dose at the right time and via the right route; that you have the right and clear documentation, the right effectiveness of the drug – that is, it has not expired – and the right allergy information recorded – in other words, your patient is not allergic to the medications being given.

Right patient: it is essential that any medication prescribed for an individual is given to the correct patient. Sadly, it is surprisingly easy to get this wrong, either through healthcare professional error, complacency or, as can be seen in George's case study at the beginning of this chapter, through service users' non-compliance. In hospital settings, name bands are commonly used to check patient identity and often include the patient's full name, date of birth and a unique hospital identity number. Some patients will not tolerate wearing a name band, however, and in some care settings the wearing of a band will be unacceptable. In such circumstances, verbal confirmation of identity may be sought, but this has its own pitfalls – for example, when dealing with young children, those who are confused, unable to speak English or have other communication challenges. Your different care settings will have developed systems to assist in correct identification, and this may include two people to confirm the right patient or photograph utilisation as examples.

Right medicine: it is also essential that as well as confirming the name of the right patient, that the right drug is administered. This seems obvious, but sometimes it is difficult to be certain from the prescription what is required. This may be due to the illegible handwriting of the prescriber, the use of unfamiliar abbreviations or the use of unclear names. As discussed in Chapter 3, a drug will have a chemical name describing its chemical composition and molecular structure, a generic name which indicates the active ingredient of the medicine and its proprietary or trade name. The use of the non-proprietary name on the prescription allows for the most cost-effective drug to be administered, but this requires you to be familiar with the medications in your service area and to know how to look up those you are unfamiliar with. Any uncertainties need to be discussed with the prescriber and, if appropriate, the pharmacist as the dispenser. It is important that abbreviations, if used, are approved and clearly understood, medicines with similar names and packaging are identified and vitally you can clearly read and understand the prescription chart you are dealing with.

Right dose: once you have ascertained that you have the correct patient and you know which drug you are to administer, you need to be certain of the correct dose. As well as being able to read this clearly, you need to be certain that what you are about to give is appropriate. It is essential to be familiar with the usual dose range of medicines in your service area and field of practice. This may be challenging, as many medicines have a variety of uses and the associated dose will vary. As mentioned in Chapter 1, aspirin as an analgesic has an acceptable higher dose than if it is being used as an antifibrinolytic, for example. Therefore, as well as the medication, you will need to know why the service user is taking it. The preparation of the medicine may additionally determine the dose, whether the drug is in a syrup or tablet form, for example, or being administered intravenously as absorption rates will vary. For example, the medication digoxin, which increases the force of contractions in the heart muscle and is commonly used for patients like George with persistent atrial fibrillation, is dispensed as a 125 microgram tablet, but is equivalent to 100 micrograms for intravenous use (BNF, 2023). Nursing associates working with children will be familiar with medicine doses prescribed according to their weight, which will require numeracy competence discussed in Chapter 5. As a rule of thumb, if your calculation or conclusion of dose required results in requiring fractions of a tablet or ridiculously large numbers, then this should give you cause to stop and reconsider both the prescription and/or the calculation. Once again, timely discussion with the prescriber and dispenser will be necessary prior to administration.

Right time: it is important that medications are given at the time stated on the prescription, or as near as possible. This is particularly important with medications denoted as critical, and your service areas will include **critical medications** within policies and procedures. One example is levodopa, a medication used to alleviate symptoms in Parkinson's disease. Strict adherence to dosage times reduces the potential for severely debilitating symptoms to reoccur for service users. Other examples will include medications, such as antibiotics, required to maintain a therapeutic level within the bloodstream. Some medicines will require to be taken with food or before mealtimes and as such will additionally require appropriate time management from you. Surveillance is also required for medications that can be given as required, pro re nata (PRN), for symptom control, outside regular dosing patterns and topical patch medications whose time management includes use over time and break periods as necessary.

Right route: medicines must always be given by the route or means of administration denoted on the prescription. You will be aware that medicines can be absorbed through being swallowed, by being placed under the skin, by being injected into a vein and so on. We will examine the procedures required for each of these administration routes later in this chapter, but for now it is important to ensure that you know which is required, as patients can become seriously ill if a medicine is given by the wrong route. This is because of the pharmacokinetics and pharmacodynamics discussed in Chapter 3. You will need to be especially vigilant for medicines that can be administered in a variety of ways to check that you are adhering to the prescriber's wishes.

Right documentation: it goes without saying in healthcare that poor documentation is a recipe for disaster. This is especially true with medicines administration. All members of the team need to be certain what drugs have been given and when. Your service areas will have clear guidance on how you complete the documentation, whether this is in paper or electronic format. You need to be clear on how to demonstrate that administration has occurred, in addition to when a medicine has been refused or not given for any reason. If you are confronted with an incomplete prescription chart with administration signatures missing, you will not know if this is a result of complacency on your predecessor's part when they forgot to sign, whether this was a result of the patient refusing their prescribed medicine, or whether there was a legitimate clinical reason for omission and your patient may not be able to explain. Whatever action you take as a result of this poor documentation could have severe consequences for your patient. Part of this complete documentation is also to ensure that medications given in a complementary health unit are clearly defined. An analgesic, like paracetamol, may have been given as part of a surgical procedure and documented within theatre notes, but not on a main prescription chart. Therefore, scrutiny of all associated paperwork is required prior to any medication administration. Remember, this chart will form part of the patient's permanent health record and as such may be used if services are called to account.

Right effectiveness (not expired): we will all have at some time rooted through our food cupboards and debated whether to eat something which is a few days past its expiry date. We base our decision on whether to consume the contents, depending on what the food substance is, how long we have had it and what it looks and smells like. This may or may not have consequences on our immediate health. We cannot afford this complacency with medicines administration, however. Medications, as chemical compositions, may well retain much of their original potency after the expiration date, but the effectiveness of the drug may decrease over time, and in some cases may render them not safe to use. Some medicines will have a short expiry date, such as prepared antibiotic mixtures where the stability of the product will change, like the antibiotic syrup prescribed for George in the case study at the beginning of the chapter. Eye drops should be discarded after a few weeks of opening as eyes are particularly sensitive to any bacteria that might get into opened eye-drop bottles. Medications that have expired need to be returned to pharmacists who can safely dispose of them. It is not acceptable to flush them into our waste-water systems.

Right allergy check: it is fundamental that we do not wish our patients harm and do not wish to administer anything that will cause them to have an adverse reaction, as explained later in this chapter. Thus, it is important to check whether our service users have any known allergies to medications or food substances. In addition, it is good practice to ask if our service users have any drug intolerances – those medications for which they are not allergic, but that cause them distressing symptoms. In these circumstances, it may be possible for an alternative to be found. Care is needed when documenting allergies, as many service users will claim an allergy for those substances they find unpleasant to take. As well as checking for allergies and intolerances, it is good practice to understand your patient's underlying and previous medical history, as some medicines you administer may cause symptoms to get worse or mask health problems all together.

Each time that a medication is given, it is suggested that you remember to do three checks. This means that you are going to do a triple check to ensure that the eight rights are present. First, remove the medication from its place of safety and check the medication label against the prescription to make sure they match. Second, before pouring or selecting the medicine, check the medicine label and prescription again. Third, before administration of the medication, check once more that it is correct.

While all these steps and checks may appear laborious, by routinely sticking to this regimen, it will be almost impossible for you to be involved in a medication error. This is assuming that you have not made a drugs calculation error. Help to ensure that you are proficient with drug calculations will be discussed in Chapter 5. If you are involved in an error, you will remember that we previously introduced the importance of an open culture or duty of candour (NMC, 2022), with the intention that healthcare providers are open and honest with their service users. This fosters an environment where safety is the priority rather than concern for individual blame. Reporting and escalation procedures in such circumstances will be discussed later in this chapter.

All healthcare environments will have a written policy on medicines management that consider legal and professional requirements. All staff will be required to read it and comply with its contents. As a nursing associate, you will be working in a variety of healthcare environments, as well as service users' own homes. Thus, the wearing of identification bracelets, the format the medication is dispensed in and where drugs are being stored will all vary. Safe administration will require vigilance, therefore, to minimise the potential for harm. It is also your responsibility to assess the patient's condition prior to administration to ensure the appropriateness of administration. If this assessment indicates that a medicine is not appropriate at this time or a contraindication is noted, then you will need to refrain from administration and contact the prescriber in a timely fashion. For example, the drug digoxin, which increases the force of contractions in the heart muscle, should not be given if the patient's pulse rate is below 60 beats a minute (BNF, 2023), as we discovered with George in the case study at the beginning of the chapter.

As employers will maintain local policies, they will specify what medicines and which routes of administration are within the parameters of your practice. This will include any safety critical medicines and those identified as controlled under the Misuse of Drugs legislation. Within all routes of medicine administration, there exist medicines that carry a higher risk of harm, sometimes referred to as **safety critical medicines** (HEE, 2017). Examples of these may include methotrexate, warfarin, insulin, digoxin lithium, opioids and medicines used outside their authorisation or recently licensed (black triangle drugs); see Chapter 1 to refresh your memory on drug licensing. Your employing organisation will define your role in their administration to promote a patient safety culture. Thus, they will define the acceptable routes of administration, the threshold standard of competence, necessary education and lines of delegation and accountability (HEE, 2017).

As you discovered when reading George's case study, we commonly encounter challenges associated with medicines administration. Now that you have explored the ethical and procedural considerations for safe medicines administration, complete Activity 4.1 to test your understanding.

Activity 4.1   Critical thinking

Reviewing the case study at the beginning of this chapter, consider George taking the oral morphine solution to control pain and aid sleep, the omission of the prescribed digoxin and the role of the nursing associate in medicines administration. Answer the following questions to develop your critical thinking abilities.

- George has confided taking his wife's oral morphine solution to control his pain and help him sleep. What are the issues regarding consent for medication administration?
- How do the 'rights' of administration apply in this situation?
- What documentation is required for George?

An outline answer is given at the end of this chapter.

Now that we have reviewed the ethical and safety critical steps to medicines administration, we can consider the variety of routes a medicine can be administered and the implications for healthcare providers and the service user.

As you discovered when reading George's case study, we use a variety of forms of medications and routes of administration. Activity 4.2 asks you to reflect on your current knowledge of what routes are commonly used and the implications for service users.

Activity 4.2   Reflection

Think of an example when you have observed or been involved with medicines administration.

- What route of administration was used, and what advantages and disadvantages can you think of for the various routes of administration?
- What were the service users' experiences with the differing routes?

As this answer is based on your own observation and reflection, there is no outline answer at the end of this chapter.

You may wish to discuss this reflection with colleagues and retain the information in a personal portfolio.

Having thought about your observations regarding medicines administration, let us consider the different routes that medicines can be administered, the implications for patients and some of the specific procedural requirements to take into consideration.

Routes of administration

As you will have observed in your practice areas, there are a number of ways that medicines can get into the body: via the gastrointestinal tract, known as **enteral**; taken into the body in a manner other than through the digestive canal, known as **parenteral**, which is often through the intravenous or injection route and **topically**, through the skin, or elsewhere in the body where the medication is directly applied to the area required. A variety of sites and methods can be used, including oral, rectal, vaginal, respiratory, intradermal injection, topical or transdermal, intravenous, intrathecal or epidural, and subcutaneous.

The aim of drug treatment is to deliver the optimal amount of the medication to the area where it is required with a minimum of harm, and this usually includes having the therapeutic level or concentration of the drug where it is needed as quickly as possible. The quickest route to achieve this therapeutic dose is intravenous, as it ensures that the medicine is delivered directly into the bloodstream. The way in which a drug is administered will affect not only the procedural technique for administration but also the rate and extent of absorption. This was discussed in Chapter 3 when the pharmacology of medicines was described. Each route of administration additionally has its advantages and disadvantages.

Oral: the most common route and it is usually the safest, most convenient and acceptable to service users, and also the least expensive. Oral preparations are available in different forms, including tablets, capsules suspensions or syrups, and can be tailored to different clinical circumstances – for example, as a slow-release preparation to allow a single dose to be effective over a longer period, mixed with a pleasant flavoured syrup to make taking it more palatable for children or as a suspension for those patients unable to take tablets. However, all these formulations can only be given if the service user is conscious and able to swallow. Some medication cannot be given orally, if, for example, it would be destroyed by the action of digestion, or if there was a clinical reason why this route would be unavailable, in which case another formulation would need to be sought. In addition, as you discovered in Chapter 3, everything that is absorbed from the intestine is carried in the bloodstream to the liver as the prime site of metabolism, which can result in a large amount of the drug being metabolised and thus not available at its intended source.

Intravenous: medication is administered directly into the bloodstream, usually through a needle or cannula. The most common drugs given via this route include replacement fluids and electrolytes, antibiotics and analgesics. Medicines delivered this way have a rapid onset of action, are more reliable as accurate titrated doses may be given and may be used when administration is required quickly, and other routes are not available. However, they need to be administered by appropriately trained individuals, are time-consuming to attend to, are usually more costly and are often unpopular with patients. In addition, there is a risk of toxicity or accidental overdoses and infection, as you are bypassing the skin's natural defences. The risk of shock, anaphylaxis and local trauma, including phlebitis, haematoma and surrounding tissue infiltration must also be considered. As a nursing associate, you may not be administering medicines via this route. However, as a member of the multidisciplinary team, you will certainly come across and be involved in the care of patients having this route of administration in your service areas. Familiarity with the risks, escalation routes and your role requirements are essential.

Intramuscular: the route of administration whereby the medicine is injected into the densest part of the selected muscle. A smaller range of drugs are given via this route, and examples include antipsychotics and immunisations. Several sites can be used, including mid-deltoid, dorsogluteal and ventrogluteal, with the drug onset of action being dependent on the blood flow at the injection site. Therefore, the elderly with decreased muscle mass and hot or cold environments can affect the effectiveness of the administration. The intramuscular route is particularly useful for drugs that are not readily soluble and, when delivered in a suspension form, can produce a slow sustained release of medication. This reservoir of drug can create a long-lasting effect and is useful, for example, for service users having antipsychotic **depot** medication.

Subcutaneous: injections given via this route are administered into the fat layer just under the skin. This relatively simple administration route can be used for medicines that require predictable and very specific dosing like insulins, and as they require very little training can be taught easily to patients and their families. Following administration, the medicine enters the capillary bloodstream through diffusion or filtration, which we explored in Chapter 3, providing slow absorption. Repeated injections at the same site may cause pain and damage to underlying tissue, however, and therefore a rotation of sites is recommended.

Topical: this route allows local absorption through the epidermis, outer layer of the skin, or external mucous membranes. Creams, lotions, ointments and pastes differ depending on whether they are water-based, prepared in a grease base or have a high solid content. This route allows the application of medication directly to the affected area which can avoid unwanted side effects. For example, the anti-inflammatories can be administered directly to a painful joint area with low risk of gastric irritation, which may occur if the drug was given orally. Commonly for creams, the dose is measured as a **fingertip unit (FTU)** and it is good practice not to allow these medications to touch your skin; impermeable gloves should therefore be worn. Service users need to be advised to wash their hands thoroughly after application of cream if they are applying it with ungloved hands. This unit of measurement does make it difficult to know exactly how much of a medication is being given to a patient, however. Other topical medications include eye drops administered to the mucous membrane. As with creams, accurate dosing is hard to ensure as bottles of liquid need to be inverted for administration and many service users find it difficult to self-administer. Care is additionally required to prevent cross-infection from one eye to another, and as they seldom contain preservatives or only mild antiseptics, the opened bottle is at risk of becoming contaminated even when stored in the fridge.

Transdermal: medicines are administered through a patch or plaster that contain a reservoir of the drug. This medication slowly seeps out and passes through the skin into the underlying tissue. The drug is then absorbed into the blood capillaries and enters the systemic circulation and therefore side effects are possible. Examples of transdermal medications include nicotine patches, hormone replacement therapy and analgesics like fentanyl patches. They are easy to use and many service users will self-administer. However, they can be indiscrete and some service users may find this embarrassing; they can also be affected by environmental factors, like hot weather, which may cause patients to perspire and the patch not to stick. Many service users will develop an intolerance to the adhesive properties of the patch and a local skin irritation may occur and finally patients may forget to remove old patches.

Inhalation: inhaling a drug directly into the respiratory system can be a very effective means of delivering a medicine to the tissues. It is particularly useful in treating conditions such as asthma and chronic obstructive airway disease. It is also an effective means of administering inhalation anaesthetics for surgery. These gases, powders or aerosols are rapidly absorbed and have a localised effect. While they can deliver a medicine to the lung tissue quickly to provide relief of symptoms, they are reliant on the patient using the correct technique. Patients using aerosol inhalers, known as metred dose inhalers, will usually get the best results using a spacer. Those of you working with young children may well be familiar with these devices, but it is important that all patients are counselled on technique and have a device that suits their individual needs to improve compliance.

Rectal: some medicines can be administered by placement directly in the rectum as an enema or suppository formulation and are readily absorbed. Medicines administered in this way can be for local or systemic effect – for example, aperients which are used to treat constipation, or analgesics and anticonvulsants which are used when a service user is having an epileptic fit. While this route offers the opportunity to administer medicine when other routes are unavailable, there is the potential for the drug to be lost from the rectal cavity before it has been absorbed, and many patients find the prospect of having a rectal medicine embarrassing or distressing, which can lead to refusal.

Vaginal: these can be creams or pessaries (solid pellets) inserted into the vagina for a localised effect. They are best inserted last thing at night or when the service user is resting to prevent them becoming dislodged and falling out. As with rectal medicines, some patients may find this treatment embarrassing, and dignity, privacy and comfort need to be assured.

Administration procedures

When administering any medication, it is important to follow standard hygiene and universal precautions as well as safe administration procedures. This will include the completion of the rights and checks as explored above, and the maintenance of safety, dignity, privacy and comfort. For specific routes, there are additional requirements to take into consideration.

Oral: these medications are available in different forms and can be tailored to different clinical circumstances. Dispersible tablets – those that do not completely dissolve, like soluble preparations – give a cloudy liquid for the service user to take – for example, dispersible aspirin. Granules need to be mixed with water and then consumed quite quickly before they become too thick to drink with the passage of time to drink – for example, the aperient fybogel. When administering these, it is important that the contents of the glass or container are swirled around, and the container may need to be rinsed to ensure that the patient receives the full dose of the medication, as some of the contents may stick to the cup or glass.

You will remember from Chapter 1 that it is not acceptable to open capsules, crush tablets or cut them, unless they are scored and you have the correct tablet-cutting equipment to ensure that your patient is receiving the correct dose.

For liquid medications, in the UK a standard dose is usually 5 millilitres (ml) and medicine spoons and cups are available to accurately measure the correct dose. Household teaspoons should not be used as they can hold anything from 4 to 8 ml of liquid. For children who may require more assistance or a lower volume than 5 ml, an oral syringe should be used. These are usually dispensed with the medication and are coloured so as not to be confused with regular syringes. Syrup formulations additionally may have an adaptor to fit to the bottle to use with these syringes and prevent spillage. Administering these formulations requires the syrup to be carefully introduced into the mouth cavity, never squirted directly at the back of the throat, as there is a risk of choking or inhalation.

To achieve the maximum absorption and minimal side effect, oral medication will need to be given as directed on the prescription, and this may be with, before or after food. A few examples include ibuprofen, a non-steroidal anti-inflammatory taken with food due to the potentially damaging effects on the gastrointestinal tract and oxytetracycline whose absorption is reduced if the service user consumes dairy products (BNF, 2023).

Some medications may be prescribed in a sublingual form requiring the service user to hold the medication under their tongue to allow it to dissolve; as a buccal medication, requiring the drug to be placed between the gum and the inside of the mouth, or as a spray to disperse the drug on to the mouth mucosa. These preparations allow for rapid absorption and avoid being broken down in the stomach and metabolised in the liver – for example, glyceryl trinitrate (GTN) spray, which is used to dilate coronary arteries as symptom relief for angina sufferers, which is inactive and therefore ineffective if swallowed.

Enteral: administration directly into the gastrointestinal tract when swallowing difficulties are present requires specific procedural technique and medications must be authorised to be given via the nasogastric and percutaneous endoscopic gastrostomy (PEG) route. In this circumstance, any enteral feed needs to be stopped prior to administration, the tube flushed, drugs administered separately as prescribed and then reflushed prior to feed recommencing. If you are involved in the administration of medicines via this enteral route, your service area employer will have specific policy and procedures to follow, and you should familiarise yourself with these.

Inhalation: it is important to deliver inhaled medicines into the lungs to achieve a rapid reaction and minimise adverse effects. A variety of inhalation devices exist. An **inhaler** is a metred dose device that will allow a specific amount of the drug to be delivered via a mouthpiece. Service users need to be taught the correct technique for self-administration. The inhaler requires shaking and the mouthpiece cover to be removed. The patient then needs to breathe out gently, place the mouthpiece in their mouth, ensuring that their lips seal around the device. As they slowly breathe in, the cannister is pressed down while they continue to breathe slowly, deeply and steadily. They should then hold their breath for 10 seconds if this is comfortable. If a second dose is required, the technique is repeated after approximately 30 seconds. Recommended for all who use an inhaler is a device called a **spacer**. This large plastic device has a hole at one end for the mouthpiece of the inhaler to be inserted and another mouthpiece at the other end for drug administration. The spacer is designed to hold the medicine while the patient inhales and is useful for those service users who find it difficult to simultaneously compress the cannister and inhale. **Nebulisers** use compressed air to change a liquid medication into a fine mist, which can then be inhaled through a mouthpiece or mask. You will need to have the correct particle size, which is best obtained by using an air flow rate of 6–8 litres/minute.

Oxygen should be regarded as a medicine. It is available under the NHS in England and Wales as emergency oxygen, a short burst of intermittent therapy, long term or ambulatory oxygen. It is prescribed for service users who are hypoxaemic to increase alveolar oxygen tension and decrease the work of breathing (BNF, 2023). The concentration required depends on the individual and the condition being treated, as incorrect or inappropriate oxygen concentrations can have serious consequences for your patient; usually it will be prescribed to achieve a measured blood oxygen saturation level. In medical emergencies, this is usually 94–98 per cent. In some clinical situations, it will be appropriate for a lower target of 88–92 per cent for your patient to become stable. Whatever the treatment requirement, you will need to be familiar with the equipment required and the additional safety concerns for oxygen therapy. Under the NHS, oxygen may be supplied in cylinders or concentrators, with nasal cannula being preferable for long-term usage, although this mode of delivery while allowing your patient to eat and drink does not allow for accurate concentration measurement. Domiciliary, or at home, and ambulatory oxygen therapy will only be instigated for long-term use after a service user has been carefully assessed by respiratory experts. If involved with their care, you will need to ensure that the patient is fully advised of the safety concerns. Adults or children who are discharged home on oxygen will require all the necessary equipment, supplies, education and support to continue the treatment. For children, this may include training parents to use apnoea monitors and oxygen saturation monitors; everyone must be educated on the safe storage of equipment and awareness of fire risk. Smoking should not be permitted in the room or transport vehicle when oxygen therapy is in use. All practice areas will have local policies for oxygen therapy. Community services will include the provision, replacement and repair of equipment, and management and transport plans.

As with all medication administration, patient comfort and compliance are essential. This requires oxygen masks and nasal cannula to be properly positioned. To counteract the drying effect of oxygen, patients should be assisted and encouraged to increase their oral fluid intake; unless delivered at a flow rate of greater than 4 litres per minute, oxygen therapy delivered through a mask or nasal cannula does not require humidification as the air that it mixes with on inspiration contains sufficient water vapour. The use of lubricants like glycerin can moisten the lips or nasal mucosa. Paraffin-based lubricants will need to be avoided due to their flammable nature.

Injections: any medication entry that bypasses the skin as the natural defence layer has the potential to introduce micro-organisms into the body. As preventing and controlling the spread of infection underpins all aspects of nursing care, you will need to be aware of your role when preparing and administering injectable medicines. After handwashing, aseptic technique should be used to prevent contamination of syringes and needles when undertaking intramuscular or subcutaneous injection. Some subcutaneous medications for injection will be dispensed as a pre-filled syringe, and insulin should be measured and administered using specifically manufactured disposable insulin syringes that are specifically calibrated in units of insulin rather than millilitres. Chapter 5 will help you to understand these units of measurement better. In addition, you will need to check your organisation's policy regarding skin preparation for your patient prior to injection. Some will advocate the use of alcohol swabs to be used and allowed to dry for 30 seconds prior to injection. However, there is much debate regarding the effectiveness of this process and, in fact, whether this causes hardening of the skin; many employers will argue that your patient's socially clean skin is all that is required. As with all aspects of your care, you will need to adhere to your organisation's specific policy. You will also need to remember to dispose of all sharps appropriately and never to resheath a used needle for risk of needlestick injury. If you do accidentally pierce your own skin with a used needle, your employing organisation will have a procedure and reporting mechanism for you to follow.

Rectal and vaginal routes: as well as assuring dignity, privacy and comfort, these routes of administration will involve you coming into contact with bodily fluids. You will need to wear **personal protective clothing (PPE)**, with apron and gloves as a minimum.

Understanding the theory: Safe administration

At the beginning of this chapter we stated that you will need to demonstrate your safety and proficiency with medicines administration to achieve qualification, join and remain on the register. It may seem as if there has been a lot of theory here for you to read and understand, and the focus on safety may seem laborious and possibly daunting. However, you will already have been abiding by much of these safety procedures during your daily practice and in your home life without being overtly aware of it. Any occasion when you have looked at the label on a medicine to see who it has been prescribed for, or been aware of your friends' and family's allergies, and known where they keep auto-injectable medications, or checked the expiry date of a product, you have been adhering to safety procedures. These are all examples of your putting theory into practice.

Now that we have explored the ethical and safety steps when assisting our service users with taking their medications, we need to consider what can go wrong, and what your role is to respond, document and escalate the concerns in these situations.

As we discovered in Chapter 1, a medicine is a substance that exerts a pharmacological, immunological or metabolic action; therefore, as well as restoring, correcting or modifying a physiological function for preventing or treating disease, there is the potential for harm.

Adverse drug reactions

An **ADR** is any unwanted or harmful reaction that occurs after the administration of a medicine, via any route, which you can be certain has occurred directly because of the drug. These can include life-threatening occurrences or unpleasant signs and symptoms that may require further medication to alleviate. These reactions can be divided into those that are predictable as a result of excessive pharmacological effect and those that are unpredictable, often a result of an immunological response. Predictable, dose-related reactions may include the respiratory depression associated with opioids, like the oramorph being self-medicated by George in the case study at the beginning of this chapter. Unpredictable ADR may include hypersensitivity rashes or the more serious anaphylaxis, which we will discuss in detail later, as a result of an unknown intolerance to a medication. The term 'iatrogenic' describes illness caused by medical treatment, and often is a direct result of drug administration, with certain patient groups being more vulnerable than others to the effects.

Predisposing factors to ADRs include ethnicity, age and pre-existing disease. The elderly and the very young, and those patients with certain genetic factors or renal disease can have a reduced ability to eliminate medications. In addition, service users taking a variety of medications, known as polypharmacy, are at increased risk of suffering an adverse effect, as one drug may influence the effects of another, known as a **drug interaction**. In addition, some drugs are known to cause more ADRs than others. These include the antibiotics, antipsychotics, non-steroidal anti-inflammatories, lithium, diuretics, benzodiazepines, drugs with a narrow therapeutic range like warfarin, and newly licensed medicines, denoted on their labelling and within the BNF with a black triangle.

Pharmacovigilance is the term used to describe the monitoring of drug safety. Clinical drug trials establish initial safety issues and concerns, and form part of the risk and benefit analysis undertaken by the manufacturers. Before marketing, however, only the initial reactions, side effects and contraindications will have been established; the further detection and monitoring of adverse events occur once medications are in common use. The standard **yellow card** produced by the Medicine and Healthcare products Regulatory Agency (MHRA), used by healthcare professionals and the version available for the general public, allows the reporting of suspected ADRs. If a pattern of side effects emerges, the MHRA informs healthcare professionals of the findings and any action needed. Healthcare professionals are expected to report all suspected ADRs for new medicines and the black triangle drugs, which are being closely monitored. Activity 4.3 explores this further.

Activity 4.3   Work-based learning

What are the main points about adverse drug reactions which are listed on the MHRA website, www.yellowcard.gov.uk, or within the adverse reactions to drugs pages and back leaf, yellow pages in the *British National Formulary*?

As this answer is based on your own exploration, there is no outline answer at the end of this chapter.

Now that you have reviewed the unwanted effects a medication can have on your service user and the procedure for reporting adverse reactions, we can explore the effects that medications can have on each other.

Drug interaction

A drug interaction describes the situation where the potency, or effectiveness, of the medication is affected by another substance. The medication may be prevented from performing as expected by another medication, by food and drink or other substances, and by specific behaviour, like high alcohol intake or smoking. The BNF classifies drug interactions as either pharmacodynamic or pharmacokinetic in nature. Pharmacodynamic interactions occur with drugs that have a similar mode of action – for example, diazepam from the benzodiazepine group and alcohol. Both these substances cause central nervous system depression and will have a combined effect. Pharmaco-kinetic interactions occur when the absorption, distribution, metabolism or excretion of one sub-stance is affected by another. Review Chapter 3 to refresh your memory on these terms. An example here might be a low-dose oestrogen oral contraceptive pill and antibiotics as the antibiotic reduces the gut bacteria that would normally induce liver enzyme activity (BNF, 2023); thus, absorption is reduced and potentially increases the risk of an unwanted pregnancy. Another example is clozapine used for the treatment of schizophrenia, which should not be given with cranberry or grapefruit juice, and which requires very careful dose adjustment if the service user changes their smoking habits. Smoking requires the patient's liver to produce isoenzymes to metabolise the harmful chemicals in a cigarette. However, this overabundance of enzymes will also metabolise the psy-chotropic agents prescribed for many mental health conditions. Heavy smokers may experience sub-therapeutic levels of the medication, but if they quit smoking while continuing with the medication regimen, they may then have increased plasma levels and risk toxicity. The BNF publication classifies interactions that are potentially serious, often described as a **contraindication**, and document where simultaneous administration of two medications should be avoided.

As with ADRs, some individuals, including older people, children and the mentally ill, may be at higher risk of susceptibility to drug interactions. Recognising the potential factors is challenging and requires the vigilance of all members of the multidisciplinary team, with the knowledge and experience of the pharmacist being essential. You will be aware that in some areas of medicine, research is scarce as it relies on compliant persons in addition to excluding many patient groups such as the very young, so not all drug interactions have been docu-mented. In addition, there may be problems obtaining truthful and accurate histories and experiences from some service users regarding medication use, particularly if interactions are the result of illicit substance misuse or risky behaviour.

As a nursing associate, you will be well placed to observe your patients and communicate concerns regarding allergies, drug sensitivity, side effects, contraindications and adverse reactions with the prescribers when managing medicines, and will use the BNF data to assist you. Activity 4.4 explores this further.

Activity 4.4   Work-based learning

What are the interactions denoted in the BNF, Appendix 1, for medications you see regularly administered within your role?

This answer is based on your own exploration. There is just one search result at the end of this chapter as an example.

While the pharmaceutical industry makes every effort to ensure the safety of medicines prior to marketing and the MHRA yellow card scheme assists to gather more data, there are some chemical substances that are known to have detrimental effects to health. Some influence foetal development causing abnormalities known as **teratogenesis**. These substances may cause abnormalities if taken in the first trimester, or first few months of pregnancy, as most medications can pass through the placenta. Care is needed therefore for the prescribing and administering of medications to pregnant women, and generally drugs should only be prescribed if the expected benefit to the mother is thought to be greater than the risk to the foetus. For many drugs, there is insufficient evidence to provide definitive guidance for prescribers for breast-feeding mothers. The amount of drug transferred in breast milk is rarely sufficient to produce a discernible effect (BNF, 2023). However, the guidance remains that only essential drugs should be administered to a mother during breast feeding. Rarely, drug-induced tumours can occur, known as **carcinogenesis**. Why these occur is largely unknown, but some medications are associated with a higher risk of lymphomas and leukaemias as they are gene toxic.

Now that you understand the terms 'adverse drug reactions' and 'drug interactions' and can recognise your service users who may be at an increased risk of iatrogenic effects, we need to explore the **hypersensitive** reactions to medications and how patients suffering an allergic reaction are cared for.

Hypersensitive reactions to medications are a result of an immune response to either the drug chemical itself or a product of its metabolism, called a metabolite. The substance forms an antigen that induces the body to produce antibodies and so trigger an immune response. This response can be mildly unpleasant like an itchy rash or a more serious airway obstruction and collapse.

Anaphylaxis

Anaphylaxis is a severe and potentially life-threatening reaction to a trigger. It can present with many different symptoms which usually develop quickly over a few minutes. The most common symptoms occur in the skin, respiratory cardiovascular and gastrointestinal system. It is associated with low blood pressure and difficulty in breathing and constitutes a **medical emergency**. The most common medicines to trigger anaphylaxis are antibiotics, aspirin, ibuprofen and other analgesics.

Anaphylaxis treatment

The Resuscitation Council (UK) issues guidelines for the treatment and management of anaphylaxis. It describes the recognition and treatment of an anaphylactic reaction, including the delivery of drugs for treatment. It includes the clinical guidance from NICE.

Treatment is based on basic life-support principles using the airway, breathing, circulation, disability and exposure (ABCDE) (Resuscitation Council (UK), 2021a, 2021b) approach to assess and treat. As a nursing associate, you will need to:

- call for help immediately;
- treat the greatest threat to life first – this may require CPR (cardiopulmonary resuscitation) in the absence of life signs;
- administer adrenaline therapy as first-line treatment in the anterolateral thigh and repeat the dose in five minutes if problems persist;
- ensure appropriate follow-up and on-going care (follow the NICE guideline (National Institute for Health and Care Excellence, 2020) for assessment and referral).

In healthcare settings you will need to be aware of where to find the Resuscitation Council algorithm (Resuscitation Council (UK), 2021a, 2021b) (see Figure 4.1) and resuscitation equipment quickly. Some organisations will have pre-prepared anaphylaxis kits that contain all the medication and equipment you will need for initial resuscitation in the event of an anaphylaxis episode. These should be present prior to the administration of high-risk treatments like blood transfusions and for immunisation clinics where previous patient response to a medication cannot be ascertained.

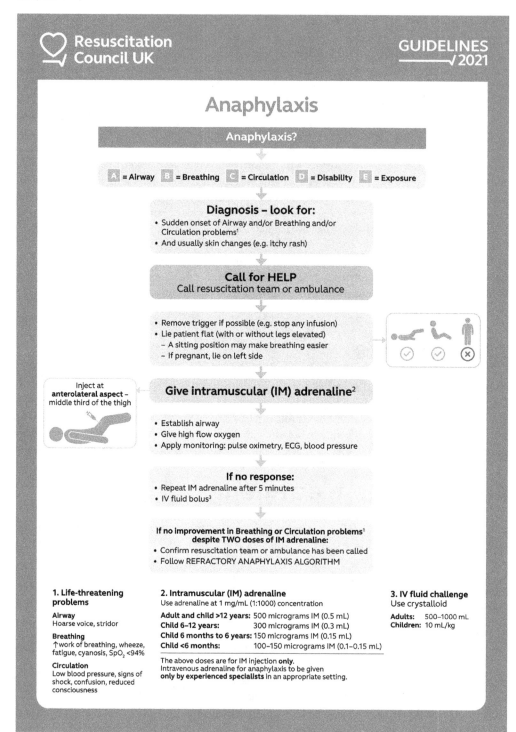

Figure 4.1 UK Resuscitation Council algorithm, 2021

Source: Produced with the kind permission of the Resuscitation Council (UK).

For those of you working with children, it is acceptable in an emergency to use length-based estimates for weight using a measurement tape device, such as the Broselow or PAWPER paediatric emergency tape. This is a long strip of laminated paper that looks like a tape measure with different coloured sections that correspond to the child's height. This tape provides all the information required, including drug dosage for emergency resuscitation of a child up to 36 kilograms.

Now that you have worked through this chapter and have explored the ethical and procedural issues associated with safe medicines administration, take some time to reflect on what you have learnt, which will allow you to apply it to your practice. Activity 4.5 will help you with this.

Activity 4.5   Reflection

- How can you define consent, concordance and covert medicines administration?
- What is your role in assuring the ethical and safe administration of medicines?
- What are the different routes of medicines administration available and what implications do these have for you as a nursing associate and your service user?
- How do you define an adverse drug reaction and a drug interaction, and how will you respond in the event of anaphylaxis?

There are no sample answers to these questions. Where you are not confident in your knowledge of a topic, you may find it necessary to reread sections of this chapter or view the further reading and websites listed at the end of this chapter to assist you. Information for questions 1 and 2 can be found in the section above on patients' rights: ethical considerations; for question 3 in the routes of administration section and for question 4 in the last section of this chapter.

You have now had the chance to reflect on the contents of this chapter and, as you can see from the summary below, that you have in fact explored a large amount of theory and been able to link this to your own practice.

Chapter summary

As you have discovered from this chapter, healthcare professionals have various ethical and safety critical responsibilities to ensure the safe administration of medicines. This chapter has outlined the service users' rights to discuss, understand and choose treatment regimens in order to promote their compliance and agreement, ensuring their consent, concordance and capacity to comply with medicines regimens. This chapter has outlined the eight steps that should be taken to ensure safe medicines administration, commonly referred to as the 'rights' of medicines administration, and described the three checks necessary for safety. It has discussed the various routes of administration and specific administration procedures. In addition, it has defined ADRs, drug interactions and anaphylaxis and its treatment.

The activities included in this chapter have invited you to consider your role in obtaining consent to treatment and asked you to reflect on the maximum benefit with the minimum of risk for medication regimes. They have required you to reflect on safe administration for the various routes and asked you to review the yellow card reporting requirements of your role. In addition, you have been asked to define an ADR a drug interaction and explore how you would respond in the event of anaphylaxis.

Activities: Brief outline answers

Activity 4.1: Critical thinking (page 60)

The healthcare team providing care for George need to ensure that he fully understands his health conditions and the treatment regimen advised for his care with a full and honest disclosure of the benefits and risks. In order to fulfil the safe taking of his medications, the 'rights' of administration will include ensuring that he only takes those medicines prescribed for him if it is appropriate to his current health state to do so. As a responsive nursing associate, you would need to discuss George's new symptom of pain and liaise with his doctor for a prescription for an appropriate analgesic to manage this. You would need to ensure that those medications that were omitted on clinical grounds were clearly documented with the reason for omission, as well as George's new symptoms of pain being documented in his health records. The RPS (2023) states that registered healthcare professionals who administer medicines are responsible for their actions, non-actions and omissions, and they must exercise professional judgement at all times.

Activity 4.4: Work-based learning (page 68)

As an example of an interaction denoted in the BNF, Appendix 1: *Paracetamol:* anticoagulants: prolonged regular use of paracetamol possibly enhances anticoagulant effect of coumarins. Antiepileptics: metabolism of paracetamol possibly accelerated by carbamazepine. Cytotoxics: paracetamol possibly inhibits metabolism of intravenous busulfan. Lipid-regulating drugs: absorption of paracetamol reduced by colestyramine. Metoclopramide: rate of absorption of paracetamol increased by metoclopramide.

Further reading

To better understand patients' rights and the ethical considerations for medicines management, the following titles may be helpful.

Blair, K (2011) *Medicines Management in Children's Nursing.* London: SAGE.

This book provides an overview of issues surrounding medicines management for those caring for children.

Mutsatsa, S (2021) *Medicines Management in Mental Health Nursing* (3rd edn). (Transforming Nursing Practice Series)

This text provides underpinning knowledge on psychotropic medications and some of their potential interactions as well as medicines management issues in mental healthcare.

National Institute for Health and Care Excellence (2019a) Giving medicines covertly.

This document outlines best practice guidance on the covert administration of medicines and provides further information on Managing medicines in care homes (SC1), Managing medicines for adults receiving social care in the community (NG67), Decision-making and mental capacity (NG108) and Care Quality Commission advice.

National Institute for Health and Care Excellence (2015) Guideline NG5. Medicines optimisation: the safe and effective use of medicines to enable the best possible outcomes.

This document discusses safe and effective use of medicines in health and social care for people taking one or more medicines. It aims to ensure that medicines provide the greatest possible benefit to people by encouraging medicines reconciliation, medication review and the use of patient decision aids.

PresQUIPP (2022). *Bulletin 269: Care homes - covert administration.*

This document explores best practice guidance on the covert administration of medicines.

To better understand the 'rights', routes and procedures for medicines administration, adverse drug reactions (ADRs), drug interactions and anaphylaxis, the following titles may be helpful.

Downie, G, Mackenzie, J and Williams, A (2008) *Pharmacology and Medicines Management for Nurses* (4th edn). Edinburgh: Churchill Livingstone.

Chapter 4 in this book will assist you to understand the different medicines administration routes and the specific procedural skills required. Chapter 10 explains different types of adverse reactions, presentation of symptoms and treatment regimes.

Resuscitation Council (UK) (2021) Emergency treatment of anaphylactic reactions: Guidelines for healthcare providers Available at https://www.resus.org.uk/library/additional-guidance/guidance-anaphylaxis/emergency-treatment.

This resource offers evidence-based guidance on the treatment algorithms for patients requiring emergency treatment for anaphylaxis.

Useful websites

The following websites are useful resources to aid your understanding.

British National Formulary: www.bnf.org

British National Formulary for Children: https://bnfc.nice.org.uk/

This website provides an overview of drug management of common conditions together with details of the medicines used. It includes latest information from clinical literature, regulatory authorities and professional bodies.

Medicines and Healthcare Products Regulatory Agency: www.mhra.gov.uk

Access to this website enables you to view and understand the work of the Medicines and Healthcare products Regulatory Agency, allowing you to report adverse medicine reactions through their yellow card scheme.

National Institute for Health and Clinical Excellence: www.nice.org.uk

This is the website of the National Institute for Health and Clinical Excellence.

Patient: www.patient.co.uk/dils.asp

Medicines information leaflets for service users are available from this website.

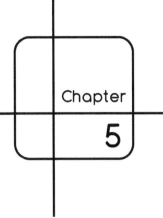

Numeracy skills for drug calculations

Chapter aims

After reading this chapter, you will be able to:

- understand the mathematical principles that provide the underlying theory to ensure accurate calculation and consequent safe administration of medicines. This will include revision of basic numeracy, conversion of units of measurement and understanding of mathematical formulas to accurately calculate medication;
- demonstrate competence in numeracy by calculating a variety of drug doses and care-related mathematical problems;
- recognise the adverse consequences of inaccurate numeracy for drug administration and understand reporting mechanisms and processes to follow if a medication error occurs.

Introduction

Case study: Lucy

You are a nursing associate working on the Children's Assessment Unit. It is over the Christmas period and the unit is short-staffed and very busy as there is an overflow of patients from A&E. This has meant that you are delayed in completing the medication round. One of your patients is an 8-year-old child called Lucy. She has been admitted due to croup. She has been prescribed dexamethasone oral solution 150 micrograms/kg as a single dose to help manage her symptoms. The oral solution in stock is 2mg/5ml. She was weighed on admission at 62 pounds. You calculate the total dose required to be 23ml, but decide to check with a colleague as the largest measure is normally 20ml. Your colleague checks your calculation and informs you that you have forgotten to convert Lucy's weight from pounds to kilograms. The correct dose should be 10.5ml. If this error had not been identified, Lucy would have been given more than double the prescribed dose.

Lucy's case study highlights the importance of having a good understanding of the key principles of general numeracy as well as drug calculation formulas to ensure patient safety. Being able to convert units of measurement correctly is essential to prevent avoidable mistakes such as this. It is also a reminder to use common sense with drug calculations and consider if the answer is practical and logical. Always double-check answers that involve excessively large numbers of tablets or volumes of solution. Recommended doses can be checked using the *British National Formulary* (BNF), and checking with another member of staff also reduces the risk of making an error. The Royal Pharmaceutical Society (RPS) (2023) advise that *any calculations needed are double-checked where practicable by a second person and uncertainties are raised with the prescriber or a pharmacy professional*. We will look in more depth at Lucy's case study as we explore different drug calculations for practice.

It is well established that numeracy and drug calculations can be a source of anxiety and worry to both trainee and qualified healthcare professionals. So, if you have a fear of maths, you are not alone. This is largely because the implications of getting it wrong can be fatal for patients, which is a big responsibility. Confidence in this skill is crucial to ensure patient safety and prevent avoidable risks to patients. This comes with experience, which is why this chapter provides plenty of clinically relevant examples for you to practise your numeracy skills and gain confidence in this area. As this is a common area of concern for health professionals, it is important that we support each other in practice to improve these skills through building a culture of safety checking.

The chapter will include an overview of basic numeracy skills, which can act as a refresher. This will ensure that you have a firm foundation to build on to be able to tackle more complicated calculations with confidence. With this in mind, you may find it helpful to work systematically through each mathematical principle as you will need to be competent in all aspects of numeracy and drug calculations that are covered in this chapter as a qualified nursing associate. This chapter is designed to be self-directed so you can review and revise aspects you feel most unsure or anxious about, as often as you like. These skills must be maintained throughout your career and form part of your continuous professional development (NMC, 2018a). Although calculators are readily available in clinical settings or on electronic devices, it is good practice to work out the mental arithmetic first or an estimation so you can check your answers against a calculator. If answers are very different, this acts as a prompt to relook at the question.

Before we begin to examine numeracy in detail, take a moment to reflect on your current understanding of mathematical principles to identify your strengths and weaknesses in this area. Activity 5.1 will help you with this.

Activity 5.1 Reflection

Consider the different numeracy topics that you require competence in as part of your role (see Table 5.1). Identify which aspects of numeracy you feel confident with and those that you find challenging or need additional revision. This will help you to prioritise your learning. Reflect on your personal numeracy competence and identify ways that you can develop this to improve your clinical practice.

As this answer is based on your own observation and reflection, there is no outline answer at the end of this chapter.

Table 5.1   The different numeracy topics and their application to practice

Numeracy topic	Application to practice	Level of confidence
Addition	Fluid balance	
	Waterlow score	
	Early warning scoring	
Subtraction	Fluid balance	
Division	BMI calculations	
	Stock management	
	Calculation of rate of enteral feed	

(Continued)

Table 5.1   (Continued)

Numeracy topic	Application to practice	Level of confidence
Multiplication	BMI calculations	
	Auditing	
Converting units of measure	Converting units available in stock to units required on the prescription	
Percentages	'MUST'	
	Auditing	
Fractions	Stock management	
Use of decimal point	Converting units of measurement	
Ratios	Adrenaline administration	
Calculating medication in tablet form	Administering tablets	
Calculating medication in liquid form	Administering injections	
	Administering oral solution	
Measuring drip rates/infusion rates	Administering enteral feeds	
Calculating dose according to weight	Paediatric doses	
	Measuring dose for high-risk medications	

Now that you have reflected on the aspects of numeracy you are relatively confident about you can continue to work your way through this chapter, recapping those elements and focussing on those you feel you need more practice on.

Mathematical principles

It is important to be familiar with basic numeracy signs and symbols to minimise errors in practice (see Table 5.2).

Table 5.2   The basic numeracy signs and symbols

Numeracy symbol	Meaning
$+$	Add
$-$	Subtract
$\times$	Multiply
$\div$	Divide
$=$	Equals
^{2}	Squared (multiplied by itself)
$\therefore$	Therefore

Numeracy symbol	Meaning
:	Ratio
<	Less than
>	More than

Units of measurement and conversion

The **metric system** is used across the NHS to measure weight, height and volume of medications using grams, metres and litres. There are a range of different units to allow the measurement of small and large items. Table 5.3 lists these and also shows the abbreviations for the units most commonly used in clinical practice.

Table 5.3   The range of different units to allow the measurement of small and large items

Metric unit	Abbreviation
Nanogram	Ng
Microgram	microgram (mcg)
Milligram	Mg
Gram	G
Kilogram	Kg
Millilitre	Ml
Litre	L

The weight and volume of medications can be measured using the following metric units:

1 kilogram = 1000 grams

1 gram = 1000 milligrams

1 milligram = 1000 micrograms

1 microgram = 1000 nanograms

1 litre = 1000 millilitres

Kilograms are used to measure large quantities, whereas nanograms are very small units of measurement. The same applies when measuring volumes. For instance, a baby who weighs 4kg at birth could also be said to weigh 4000 grams. The measurements mean exactly the same thing.

Having a range of different units prevents measures becoming excessively large or small. To avoid medication errors, it is recommended to convert measures to avoid unnecessary decimal spaces or multiples of 10. This would mean that the baby's weight should be documented as 4kg as opposed to 4000g.

To convert large to small units and vice versa, you must be familiar with the order in which they are ranked (see Figure 5.1).

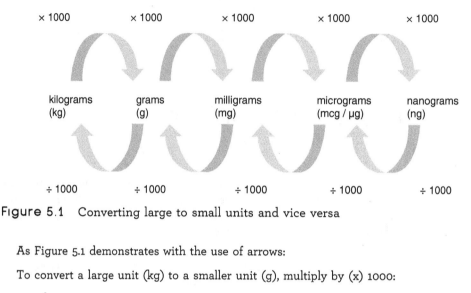

Figure 5.1   Converting large to small units and vice versa

As Figure 5.1 demonstrates with the use of arrows:

To convert a large unit (kg) to a smaller unit (g), multiply by (x) 1000:

e.g. 4kg x 1000 = 4000g

> ### Tip
>
> The smaller the unit, the larger the number will be.

If you wanted to convert a small unit (g) to a larger unit (kg), divide by (÷) 1000:

∴ 4000g ÷ 1000 = 4kg

Another example of converting a small unit to a larger one would be to convert milligrams (mg) to grams (g):

Paracetamol comes in 500mg tablets; if you want to find out what this is in grams, ÷ 1000.

500mg ÷ 1000 = 0.5g

> ### Tip
>
> Always make sure you indicate the unit of measure to avoid errors.

Multiplying and dividing by 1000 can be easily worked out by moving the decimal point backwards 3 digits when dividing and forwards 3 digits when multiplying.

For instance:

Take the number 8503 (remember this may be written as 8503.0):

8503.0 ÷ 1000 = 8.503

$$8\ 5\ 0\ 3\ .0$$

0.8503 × 1000 = 850.3

$$0.8\ 5\ 0\ 3$$

This allows you to do the conversion using mental maths, which can then be double-checked with a calculator. Have a practice with the following questions.

Activity 5.2   Calculation practice 1

1a)   0.005 × 1000 =

1b)   94773 ÷ 1000 =

1c)   0.8888 × 1000 =

1d)   94.773 × 1000 =

1e)   111 ÷ 1000 =

Answers are given at the end of this chapter.

You may need to convert more than one unit, which means you will have to do the equation more than once.

For instance, to convert 0.725kg to mg:

0.725kg × 1000 = 725g

725g × 1000 = 725,000mg

Use Figure 5.1 to help work out the following practice questions.

Activity 5.3   Calculation practice 2

2a)   Convert 3750mcg to grams.

2b)   A patient is prescribed Naproxen 1.25g. What is this in mg?

2c)   What is 0.05kg in mg?

2d)   A 1 litre bag of Nutrison ng feed is administered. What is this in ml?

2e)   There is 200ml left of the 1 litre Nutrison ng feed at the end of your shift. How many ml has the patient had?

(Continued)

(Continued)

    2f)   Your patient is prescribed 3.5mg of a medicine, but stock is only available in micrograms. What is 3.5mg in mcg?

Answers are given at the end of this chapter.

Imperial weight conversion

Consider Lucy's scenario where her weight was measured in pounds and needed to be converted into kilograms. Although there are online calculators that can work out the equation for you, to minimise errors it is best to work this out yourself, then you can check your answer afterwards. Table 5.4 includes some conversions you may need in practice. This is commonly because service users may only know their own or their children's weight in imperial as opposed to metric units. It is worth noting that most **Body Mass Index (BMI)** charts include imperial and metric units.

Table 5.4   Some conversions you may need in practice

1 pound = 0.45kg
1 kg = 2.2lb
1 stone = 6.35kg
1kg = 0.16 stone
1 metre = 3.28 feet
1 foot = 0.305 metres

Converting pounds (lb) to kilograms (kg):

1lb = 0.45kg

$\therefore$ 62lb = 0.45 × 62 = 27.9

The nearest whole number is 30kg

Alternatively, a patient is 5′ 4″ (5 feet, 4 inches) and you need this in metres to find out their BMI.

Converting feet (ft) to metres (m):

1 ft = 0.305m

$\therefore$ 5.4ft = 0.305 × 5.4 = 1.647

1.6m to 1 decimal place

Calculating the nearest whole number

Usually, you will want to round your answers off to the nearest whole number.

The rule is, if the number after the decimal point is between 0 and 4, round down; if the number is between 5 and 9, round up – for example:

9.4 rounds down to 9 as the nearest whole number

9.5 rounds up to 10 as the nearest whole number.

In some situations, you may need the number to 1 or 2 decimal places, for instance, to be able to accurately fill a syringe.

The principle remains the same: round the first decimal number up or down for 1 decimal place, or the second decimal number for 2 decimal places:

0.275ml to 1 decimal place = 0.3ml

0.275ml to 2 decimal places = 0.28ml

Activity 5.4   Calculation practice 3

5.585

3a)   Write this as a whole number.

3b)   Write this number to 1 decimal place.

3c)   Write this number to 2 decimal places.

Answers are given at the end of this chapter.

Using Table 5.4, practise the following questions.

Activity 5.5   Calculation practice 4

4a)   A service user weighs 9.5 stones. What is this to the nearest kg?

4b)   A mum wants to know how much her baby weighs in pounds and ounces. He is 3.2kg. Give your answer to 2 decimal places.

4c)   A patient asks you how much they weigh in stone (to the nearest whole number) if they are 85kg.

4d)   Convert 56lb to kg. Give your answer to the nearest whole number.

4e)   What is 6 feet in metres?

Answers are given at the end of this chapter.

Body mass index calculation

BMI charts are commonly readily available within clinical areas to calculate BMI. See Figure 5.2 for an example. There are also online BMI calculators such as the **NHS Healthy Weight Calculator**. It is good practice to calculate the weight using the formula and then check answers against the chart/online calculator.

Advice also exists to direct people to resources that give advice on how to measure their waist circumference and information to allow interpretation of waist to height ratio (NICE, 2022). The advice requires a waist circumference and height measurement to be taken in the same units.

The formula is as follows:

Weight (kg)/[height (m)]^2

If a patient weighs 82kg and is 1.78 metres tall, the first part of the equation that needs to be calculated is the height squared (^{2}). This simply means multiplying the height figure by itself, so in this case it is 1.78 $\times$ 1.78.

1.78 $\times$ 1.78 = 3.1684

$\therefore$ BMI = 82 (weight in kg) $\div$ 3.1684 (height in metres squared)

= 25.880570. . .

Rounded to the nearest whole number:

BMI 26

Now check this with the BMI chart in Figure 5.2. The answers should be the same.

You may need to convert a service user's height from feet to metres before using the formula – for instance:

Joyce is 5 feet 7 inches tall and weighs 53kg.

If 1 foot = 0.305 metres (see Table 5.4)

5' 7" in metres = 5.7 $\times$ 0.305 = 1.7385m

$\therefore$ 1.7 metres to 1 decimal place

1.7 $\times$ 1.7 (height^2) = 2.89m

53kg $\div$ 2.89m = 18.33910. . .

$\therefore$ BMI 18

This can then be checked against the BMI chart.

Weight in stones can also be converted so that the formula can be used – for example:

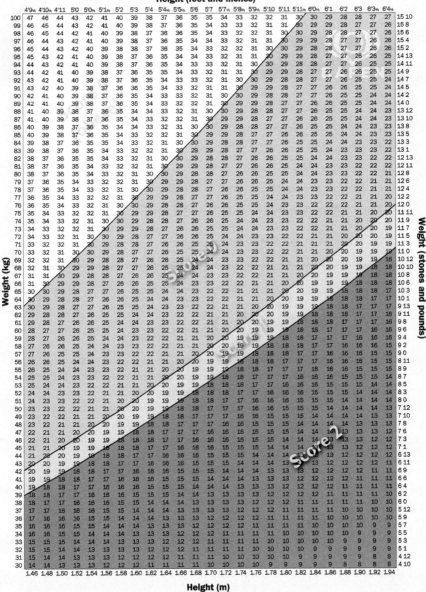

Figure 5.2 The BMI chart

Source: The BMI chart is reproduced with the kind permission of BAPEN (British Association for Parenteral and Enteral Nutrition). For further information on 'MUST', see www.bapen.org.uk

A service user weighs 7 stones 6 and is 1.5 metres tall. Calculate their BMI.

If 1 stone = 6.35kg (see Table 5.4)

7 stones 6 = 7.6 × 6.35 = **48.26kg**

His height^2: 1.5 × 1.5 = 2.25m

48.26 ÷ 2.25 = 21.4488888. . .

∴ BMI 21

Have a go at the following exercises and check your answers using the BMI chart in Figure 5.2.

Activity 5.6   Calculation practice 5

5a) Nathan is 6′ 2″ and weighs 98kg. Calculate his BMI.

5b) Julie is 1.75m tall and weighs 66kg. Calculate her BMI.

5c) Caroline weighs 88kg and is 5′ 3″. Calculate her BMI.

5d) Is Caroline categorised as obese?

5e) Nina is 1.63m and weighs 40kg. Calculate her BMI.

5e) According to Figure 5.2, what is Caroline's BMI score?

Answers are given at the end of this chapter.

Number fractions

Fractions describe parts of a whole number. This can be useful for stock acquisition to know that half of the Foley catheters have been used for example, or for auditing purposes to identify a quarter of patients are receiving antipsychotic medication.

All fractions have a numerator and a denominator. You may be familiar with the pizza analogy, so if a patient has been given a pizza which is divided into 8 equal slices, this is the denominator, the numerator is the number of slices that they have eaten, in this case 2.

$$\frac{2 \; Numerator}{8 \; Denominator}$$

This can be simplified down by dividing both the numerator and denominator by the same number.

Tip

Knowing your times tables makes it easier to simplify fractions as you know which numbers are divisible by each other – for example:

2/8 can be simplified to 1/4 as 2 and 8 are divisible by 2.

2 ÷ 2 = 1, 8 ÷ 2 = 4 = 1/4

It can be useful in practice to simplify large fractions down to make them more meaningful –for example:

50 out of 250 sharps bins have been used (50/250).

This can be simplified to 1/5 as 50 ÷ 50 = 1 and 250 ÷ 50 = 5 = 1/5

Try simplifying the following fractions.

Activity 5.7   Calculation practice 6

6a) 27/99

6b) 6/48

6c) 24/144

6d) 80/480

6e) 125/3750

Answers are given at the end of this chapter.

It is useful to be able to convert fractions, decimals and percentages as they are simply different ways of presenting the same value. Some of the most common examples are indicated in Table 5.5 to demonstrate how values can be converted.

Table 5.5   Some of the most common examples for converting fractions, decimals and percentages

Percentage	Fraction	Decimal	Percentage
1%	1/100	1 ÷ 100 = 0.01	0.01 × 100 = 1%
2%	2/100 = 1/50	1 ÷ 50 = 0.02	0.02 × 100 = 2%
5%	5/100 = 1/20	1 ÷ 20 = 0.05	0.05 × 100 = 5%
10%	10/100 = 1/10	1 ÷ 10 = 0.1	0.01 × 100 = 10%
20%	20/100 = 1/5	1 ÷ 5 = 0.2	0.2 × 100 = 20%
25%	25/100 = 1/4	1 ÷ 4 = 0.25	0.25 × 100 = 25%
50%	50/100 = 1/2	1 ÷ 2 = 0.5	0.5 × 100 = 50%
75%	75/100 = 3/4	3 ÷ 4 = 0.75	0.75 × 100 = 75%
80%	80/100 = 4/5	4 ÷ 5 = 0.8	0.8 × 100 = 80%
90%	90/100 = 9/10	9 ÷ 10 = 0.9	0.9 × 100 = 90%

Remember that the decimal place moves forward once when multiplying by 10, forward twice when multiplying by 100 and forward three spaces when multiplying by 1000 .

The decimal place moves back once when dividing by 10, back two spaces when dividing by 100 and back three spaces when dividing by 1000 .

Using the principles outlined in Table 5.5, convert the following values.

Activity 5.8   Calculation practice 7

7a)   What is 1/8 written as a decimal?

7b)   What is 0.6 written as a percentage?

7c)   What is 35% as a fraction in its simplest form?

7d)   What is 0.45 as a percentage?

7e)   What is 85% written as a fraction?

Answers are given at the end of this chapter.

Percentages

Percentages are another way of identifying a part of a whole number and, as identified in Table 5.5, can be written as a fraction out of 100. Percentages (%) are used regularly in clinical practice. The concentration of a wide range of drugs is written as %. This means that only a percentage of a drug is present in a bag of fluid, an ampoule or in a cream. One of the most common examples in clinical settings is a bag of normal saline for intravenous infusion. This is 0.9% sodium chloride (g/l) in a 1000ml bag of fluid.

To work out how much salt (sodium chloride) is in the bag of fluid, you can convert the percentage into a fraction and multiple it by the total volume. This tells you the percentage according to that particular volume.

We know that 0.9% means the same as 0.9 out of 100 (90/100).

0.9 ÷ 100 (percentage written as a fraction) × 1000 (total volume of fluid) = 9 (total concentration of drug in volume (g/l)

0.9 ÷ 100 × 1000 = **9g/l**

Therefore, there are 9 grams of salt in every litre or 1000ml of fluid.

5% dextrose (g/l) in a 1000ml bag of fluid is another example that you may see in practice.

To work out how much dextrose is in the litre bag:

5 ÷ 100 × 1000 = **50 grams of dextrose per litre or 1000ml**

If 20% of the syringe driver has been used and there was 50ml of fluid initially, how many millilitres have been used? How many are left?

To start with, find out what 20% of 50ml is:

20 ÷ 100 (20% as a fraction) × 50 (total volume) = **10ml has been used**

Therefore, 50ml (total volume) − 10ml (amount used) = **40ml left over**

The 'Malnutrition Universal Screening Tool' screen asks you to calculate the percentage of unplanned weight loss (see Figure 5.3).

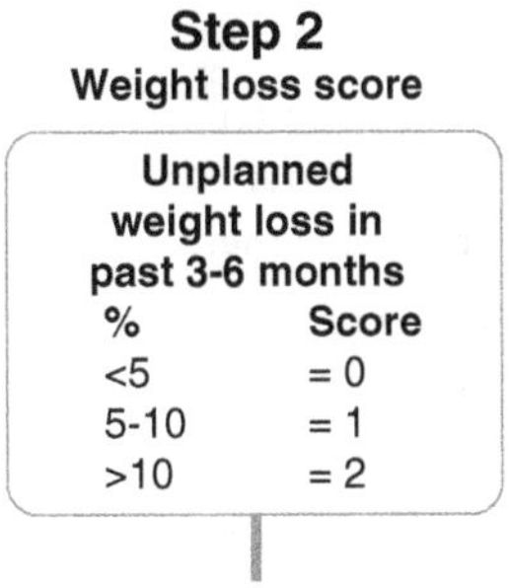

Step 2
Weight loss score

Unplanned weight loss in past 3-6 months	
%	Score
<5	= 0
5-10	= 1
>10	= 2

Figure 5.3   Part of the 'Malnutrition Universal Screening Tool' ('MUST') © BAPEN, 2011

Source: Part of the Malnutrition Universal Screening Tool is reproduced here with the kind permission of BAPEN (British Association for Parenteral and Enteral Nutrition). For further information on 'MUST', see www.bapen.org.uk

For instance, Jamil's notes indicate that she weighed 61kg at the GP surgery 4 months ago. On admission today, she weighs 57.5kg. What is her percentage of unplanned weight loss?

First, find out the amount she has lost in kg:

61 – 57.5 = Jamil has lost 3.5kg in the last 4 months.

We want to know the amount lost as a percentage of her total weight:

3.5 (amount lost) out of 61 (total weight) is 3.5 ÷ 61 = 0.057.

This figure as a percentage would be:

0.057 × 100 = 5.7%

This rounds up to 6% (as a whole number) unplanned weight loss in the last 4 months. So, Jamil would score 1 for step 2 of the 'MUST' tool (Figure 5.3).

The principles used are the same for working out the percentage of anything else in clinical practice. You may be asked to help with stock management or compiling information for monitoring or auditing purposes.

If there are 50 patients on the ward and 8 have been assessed as at risk of falls, what percentage are at risk of falls?

8 (at risk of falls) ÷ 100 (8% as a fraction) x 50 (total) = 4%

Now try the following percentage questions.

Activity 5.9   Calculation practice 8

8a)   What is 45% of 250ml?

8b)   There is 2% clotrimazole in a 20g tube of Canesten cream. How many grams of clotrimazole are there?

(Continued)

(Continued)

8c) If a patient normally weighs 75kg and has lost 4500g in the last week, what is their percentage of weight loss? Round to the nearest whole number.

8d) You are helping the ward manager with an audit. The ward currently has 50 patients, of whom 12% have an indwelling catheter; 2% have acquired an infection from their catheter. How many patients have a catheter?

8e) How many patients have acquired an infection from their catheter?

Answers are given at the end of this chapter.

Ratios

Ratios are a description of how much of one substance there is compared to another (part a: part b). Take, for instance, the ratio of a gin (a) and tonic (b). A strong gin and tonic may be in the ratio of 1:3. This means for every 1 part of gin there are 3 parts of tonic, so there is a total of 4 parts. The rule with ratios is that both part a and b must be treated the same for the ratio to remain the same. If, for instance, you want to make 3 G&Ts for friends, you will need to multiply part a by 3 as well as part b to ensure that everyone gets the same ratio of gin and tonic.

part a: $1 \times 3 = 3$ parts gin needed for 3 friends

part b: $3 \times 3 = 9$ parts tonic needed for 3 friends

If you have a single G&T at a ratio of 1:4 and the total volume is 100ml, how many millilitres are gin? To work out what 1 part is, divide the total volume by the total of both parts of the ratio (a + b):

100ml $\div$ 5 (a + b) = 20ml

gin = 20ml

Now we know what 1 part is, we can find out how much tonic there is by multiplying what one part is by part b:

20ml $\times$ 4 = 80ml

tonic = 80ml

Both elements of the ratio are liquids, so this is worked out in millilitres.

> Tip
>
> Sometimes ratios can be written in different ways. Always remember a ratio of 1:4 has a total of 5 parts, whereas if it is written as 1 in 4, this means that there are 4 total parts, one of which has the solution (drug) in it.

G&Ts do not feature much in practice, however, so here is a more relevant example.

The most common drug that is written up as a ratio in practice is adrenaline. Adrenaline is the recommended treatment for life-threatening anaphylaxis (BNF, 2023), which was discussed in Chapter 4.

For intramuscular injection, adrenaline comes in a ratio of 1 (adrenaline):1000 (solution for injection). This means that every 1ml of solution for injection contains 1mg of adrenaline (i.e: 1mg/ml or 1g in 1000ml).

The recommended dose for adults in this circumstance is 500 micrograms or 0.5mg intramuscularly (IM) (BNF, 2023).

The required dose is 0.5mg and it comes in a solution of 1mg/ml.

To work out the difference between the solution and what is prescribed, divide the stock value for part a by the prescribed value for part a ($1 \div 0.5 = 2$).

If part a has been divided by 2 to get 0.5mg, part b also needs to be divided by 2 to keep the ratio the same.

part a: 1mg $\div$ 2 = 0.5mg

part b: 1ml $\div$ 2 = 0.5ml

Therefore, 0.5ml needs to be administered.

0.25mg adrenaline is prescribed for a small child with the same ratio (1mg/ml).

1 $\div$ 0.25 = 4

If part a has been divided by 4 to get the prescribed dose, part b also needs to be divided by 4.

part a: 1mg $\div$ 4 = 0.25mg

part b: 1ml $\div$ 4 = 0.25ml

Therefore, 0.25ml needs to be administered for the child.

Adrenaline is also prescribed for other uses as 1:10,000. This is a different ratio which is a weaker solution, with less adrenaline in. This means the ratio is 0.1mg/ml.

If 1mg was prescribed intravenously, to maintain the ratio both parts would need to be treated the same:

0.1 $\div$ 1 = 0.1 (therefore part a has been divided by 0.1 to get the prescribed dose, so part b also needs to be divided by 0.1)

0.1mg $\div$ 0.1 = 1mg (desired dose)

1ml $\div$ 0.1 = 10ml (amount to be drawn up to deliver desired dose)

Therefore, 10ml would need to be administered.

As adrenaline is a solid medicinal substance mixed into a liquid, it is written as mg/ml.

Practise with the following questions.

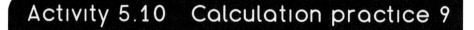

Activity 5.10   Calculation practice 9

9a)   Fluticasone cream 15g has a ratio of 1:99 (steroid:aqueous cream). How many grams of steroid are there?

9b)   Chloramphenicol eye drops 10ml are in a ratio of 1:7 (antibiotic:eye drops). How many millilitres of antibiotic are there?

9c)   How much eye-drop solution is there?

9d)   A repeat prescription is given for chloramphenicol eye drops at a ratio of 1:7, but it is in a 5ml bottle instead of a 10ml bottle. How many millilitres of antibiotic are there now? Round this to 1 decimal place.

9e)   Hydramol cream has a ratio of 1 in 8 (urea:cream). How many grams of urea would there be in a tub of 500g?

9f)   E45 has 5% urea in a 500g tub. Does E45 or Hydramol contain the most urea?

Answers are given at the end of this chapter.

Drug calculations: Administering tablets

Table 5.6   Abbreviations commonly used when administering medication

OD	Once a day
ON	Once at night
BD	Two times a day
TDS	Three times a day
QDS	Four times a day
PRN	As needed
STAT	Immediately
IM	Intramuscular
IV	Intravenous
PR	Per rectum

Some drug calculations can be calculated very easily in our head. For instance, working out how many 500mg paracetamol tablets are needed for a patient who is prescribed 1g is straightforward. Unfortunately, calculating tablets or liquids is not always very easy and can become quite complex. The good news is that there are some fail-safe numeracy equations that can be memorised to tackle any drug calculation. Using these formulas will also reduce the risk of making errors. Table 5.6 includes a range of abbreviations commonly used with calculating medication doses that you need to be familiar with.

The formula for calculating how many tablets to administer to patients is as follows.

$$\frac{\text{What you want (prescribed amount)}}{\text{What you've got (dose available in stock)}} = \text{number of tablets required}$$

For example, you have a diabetic service user who is prescribed 1.5g tablets of metformin OD. Tablets are available in 500mg. How many tablets does your patient need?

First, convert units so they are the same. As the tablets come in mg, it is best to convert to the form available in stock:

1.5g = 1500mg

What you want (1500mg) ÷ What you've got (500mg) = 3

Therefore, 3 tablets need to be given to the patient.

Your service user is prescribed 2mg risperidone due to an acute psychotic episode. The tablets in stock are 800mcg. How many tablets do they need to get the total prescribed dose?

2mg = 2000mcg

What you want (2000mcg) ÷ What you've got (800mcg) = 2.5

Therefore, 2½ tablets are needed.

Remember: always consult a pharmacist before splitting tablets as it is not always safe to do so and there may be alternative stock doses that can be ordered (see Chapter 1).

Carbamazepine 250mg is prescribed as a suppository for your patient who is having a generalised tonic-clonic seizure. The suppositories in stock are 125mg. How many does your patient need?

250mg ÷ 125mg = **2 suppositories** need to be administered.

Activity 5.11 Calculation practice 10

10a) Your patient is prescribed 3.75mg bisoprolol. Tablets are available as 1.25mg. How many tablets are needed?

10b) Nathan is prescribed ranitidine 150mg BD. In stock are 75mg tablets. How many tablets are needed?

10c) A patient is written up for 1.5mg of diazepam. There are 500mcg tablets available in stock. How many tablets need administering?

10d) Olivia is due 150mg trazadone as an antidepressant. Tablets in stock are 37.5mg. How many tablets will she need?

10e) Glycerol 4g is prescribed for constipation. Suppositories in stock are 2g. How many suppositories are needed?

(Continued)

(Continued)

10f) Catherine is written up for 75mg aspirin OD. Tablets in stock are 75mg. How many tablets will she need?

Answers are given at the end of this chapter.

Drug calculations: Administering liquids

When administering liquid medication such as oral solutions or drawing up for injections, there is a slightly different formula. This is because liquids are usually prescribed indicating the strength/concentration of the drug (usually mg or g) and the volume (usually ml or l).

$$\frac{\text{What you want (prescribed amount)}}{\text{What you've got (dose available in stock)}} \times \text{volume (ml)}$$

For instance, a patient is prescribed 5mg of oramorph solution every 4 hours. This comes as 2mg/ml.

The prescribed amount is (5mg) ÷ dose available (2mg) x volume (1ml).

5 ÷ 2 = 2.5

2.5 × 1 = 2.5ml

Remember, you are giving a fluid medication, so the unit will be in millilitres (ml).

Your patient will therefore need 2.5ml of oral solution to get the desired dose of 5mg.

Julia has been vomiting since her return from theatre. She is written up for IM cyclizine 50mg. Ampoules in stock are 50mg/1ml solution for injection.

50 ÷ 50 = 1

1 × 1 = 1ml required

Tinzaparin 3500 units is prescribed for your patient. The solution available is 10,000 units/ml. The equation remains the same, even though the unit of measure is different. It is important that you document the unit of measure carefully and use an appropriate syringe with unit measures.

3500 ÷ 10,000 × 1 = 0.35 units required

Tip

Use common sense when checking answers and make sure they are practical. The maximum amount of fluid that can be injected depends on the site of an IM injection. For instance, injections to the deltoid (shoulder muscle) should not exceed 1ml of fluid.

Activity 5.12   Calculation practice 11

11a)   100mg zuclopenthixol depot injection is prescribed for your service user. The solution for injection is available as 50mg per 1ml. How much needs to be administered?

11b)   Jason is prescribed 60mg of phenobarbital oral solution which is available as 15mg/5ml. How much needs to be given?

11c)   Your patient has been prescribed 15mg senna. The solution is 7.5mg/5ml. How much senna needs to be administered?

11d)   James is due his actrapid insulin injection. He is written up for 30 units of insulin. The stock available is 100 units/ml. How much needs to be administered?

11e)   Pethidine is available in stock as 100mg/2ml ampoules. Your patient is prescribed 75mg IM every 4 hours. How much needs to be administered?

11f)   Kate is prescribed 40mg enoxaparin sodium SC as post-surgery prophylaxis of deep vein thrombosis. Solution is available in stock as 20mg/0.2ml. How much needs to be administered?

Answers are given at the end of this chapter.

Calculations according to weight

On occasion, dosages need to be calculated according to the patient's weight. This happens frequently within the field of paediatrics as weight and size can dramatically alter during childhood. Pharmacokinetics and dynamics – that is, the effect medication has on the body and the impact the body has on medication alters throughout the lifespan (see Chapter 3). This means that in certain circumstances, such as in paediatrics, with certain elderly patients or with potent medications, standard doses are not accurate enough and individualised doses are required. For instance, IV heparin is calculated by weight as this is a high-risk medication, the dose of this anticoagulant must be accurate to reach a therapeutic dose that avoids both the risks of bleeding and the blood clotting.

The formula for calculating dose according to weight is as follows:

$$\text{Dose per kg x weight (kg)} = \text{personalised patient dose}$$

Let us consider Lucy's situation again. She is 8 years old and weighs 62 pounds. For the formula to be valid, the dose must be in kilograms (kg). Lucy's case study demonstrated the significance of working in the correct unit of measure. So first, we need to convert her weight from pounds to kilograms:

1lb = 0.45kg

62lb = 0.45 × 64 = 27.9 (28 is the nearest whole number).

So we now know that Lucy weighs **28kg**

∴ the personalised patient dose =

150 micrograms (dose per kg) × 28 (weight in kg) = 4200 micrograms or **4.2mg***

*As identified earlier, it is best to convert to the same unit of measure that is in stock so that it can be easily administered.

As the oral solution available is 2mg/5ml, we now need to work out how much to administer using the equation for administering liquids:

4.2mg (what you want) ÷ 2mg (what you've got) × 5ml (volume).

∴ 4.2 ÷ 2 × 5 = 10.5ml

Therefore, the personalised dose that needs to be administered to Lucy is 10.5ml.

Another example of a calculation according to weight is as follows:

IV erythromycin is prescribed as 6.25mg/kg every 6 hours. Your patient weighs 56kg.

To work out this equation, you simply need to multiply the dose by the patient's weight:

6.25 × 56 = 3500mg or 3.5g needs to be administered to this particular patient every 6 hours.

Although administering IV medication is not currently within the skills annexe for most nursing associates, you may be asked to check IV drug calculations with another healthcare professional. Therefore, it is important that you understand the theory. As guidance differs according to different Trust, please ensure you follow Trust policy and guidance in relation to administration of medication at all times.

A patient is due their fragmin injection. He needs 120 units/kg every 12 hours. The solution for injection comes as 10,000 units/4ml. He is 50kg. Using the equation for calculating liquids, we can work out how many units need to be administered:

120 (dose per kg) x 50 (patient's weight) = 6000 units needed every 12 hours

6000 units (what we want) ÷ 10,000 units (what we've got) x 4ml (volume) = total to administer

6000 ÷ 10,000 × 4 = 2.4ml every 12 hours

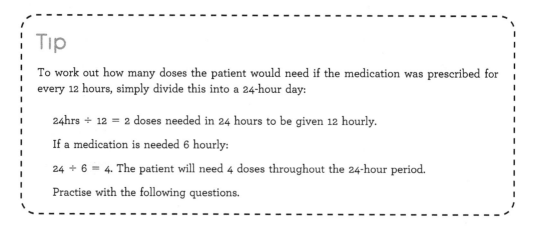

Tip

To work out how many doses the patient would need if the medication was prescribed for every 12 hours, simply divide this into a 24-hour day:

24hrs ÷ 12 = 2 doses needed in 24 hours to be given 12 hourly.

If a medication is needed 6 hourly:

24 ÷ 6 = 4. The patient will need 4 doses throughout the 24-hour period.

Practise with the following questions.

Activity 5.13   Calculation practice 12

12a) Jenna is prescribed gentamycin 3mg/kg daily, in 3 divided doses. She is 45kg. This comes in 5mg/ml solution for injection. Calculate the total daily dose needed for Jenna.

12b) Calculate the dose she will need if it is divided into 3 doses in a day.

12c) Calculate the volume that needs to be administered for each individual dose.

12d) Caden is prescribed co-amoxiclav 30mg/kg every 8 hours. Stock is available in 125mg/5ml. If he weighs 15kg, what dose will he need and how many times a day.

12e) Calculate how many millilitres need to be administered for each dose.

12f) Calculate the total daily dose of co-amoxiclav that Caden will have in a day.

Answers are given at the end of this chapter.

Drug calculations for infusion rates

As a nursing associate you may be asked to check drug calculations for IV infusions with another healthcare professional, so the formula for drip rates and IV infusions will be discussed briefly. Infusion rates also relate to the calculation and administration of enteral feeds, which is part of the NA skills annexe.

The safest way to administer IV fluids and medication is through an infusion pump as this administers a continuous flow at the exact rate entered into the device (ml/hour). Infusion pumps bleep if the line is occluded and not flowing correctly, although this can be a source of great irritation to both patients and staff alike. Without this function, occlusions to the line may be missed, which has a knock-on effect to the amount of drug being administered. Smart infusion pumps are also able to reduce medication errors by having a drug library so that rates cannot exceed minimum or maximum doses for that medication.

Drop rate

For certain infusions, where the patient and drug are considered low risk, an infusion pump may not be used and fluids instead infuse via gravity. This means that fluid flows through the giving set and the rate of infusion is set manually using the roller clamp to control the number of drops that filter through the drip chamber. The formula to calculate the number of drops that go through the drip filter per minute is outlined below.

$$\frac{\text{Volume to be infused (ml)} \times \text{drop factor (drops/ml)}}{\text{Time (mins)}} = \text{drops per minute}$$

The drop factor depends on the type of giving set that is being used:

- A regular giving set has a drop factor of 20 drops per ml.
- A blood-giving set has a drop factor of 15 drops per ml.

Drop factors on giving sets vary as the drip chamber can vary in size and length. Blood-giving sets also have a filter to enable a consistent flow. Always check the packaging on the bag of the giving set, as this will indicate what the drop factor is.

A patient is prescribed sodium chloride 0.9% 1000ml over 8 hours. A regular giving set will be used:

1000ml (volume to be infused) × 20 (drop factor) = 10,000 drops

The time in hours is 8. To convert this to minutes, multiply by 60: 8 × 60 = 480 minutes

10,000 ÷ 480 (time in minutes) = 41.66666 drops per minute

Drops can only be measured as whole numbers, so **42 drops per minute** will need to flow through the drip chamber.

IV paracetamol 100ml solution for infusion is prescribed over 30 minutes using a normal giving set.

100ml (volume to be infused) × 20 (drop factor) = 1000 drops

1000 ÷ 30 = 66.66666

∴ **67 drops per minute**

Flow rate

If an infusion pump is used, the formula and calculation are slightly different.

Let's take the first example again. The registered nurse needs to administer 1000ml 0.9% sodium chloride infusion over 8 hours. Infusion pumps administer fluid according to how many millilitres are needed to be infused every hour. To work this out:

Total volume required ÷ time to infuse (hours) = ml per hour required (flow rate)

1000 (volume) ÷ 8 (time in hours) = **125ml per hour** (flow rate)

This means that every hour for 8 hours the patient will receive 125ml.

You may be asked to set up an infusion for an ng feed. Nutricia advanced 1000ml ng feed needs to be administered over 12 hours. To work out how many ml per hour the patient needs, the same equation can be used:

1000 (volume) ÷ 12 (time) = 83.333333ml per hour

∴ flow rate = **83ml per hour** to the nearest whole number

Use the equation to calculate the following questions.

Activity 5.14   Calculation practice 13

13a) 500ml Nutrison multifibre feed over 5 hours is written up for your patient on a PEG feed. Calculate the flow rate for the patient.

13b) The district nurse asks you to double-check the infusion rate she has calculated for a palliative care patient while you are also at the patient's home. The patient has been prescribed morphine sulphate 20mg at a concentration of 1mg/ml over 24 hours. If the total volume is 20ml, calculate the correct flow rate for the patient. Give your answer to 1 decimal space.

13c) You are asked to check the drip rate for a patient who has been prescribed 1 litre of Hartmann's IV fluids over 6 hours. A regular giving set will be used. Give your answer to the nearest whole number.

13d) Janet is due her ng feed. She is prescribed 1500ml over 12 hours. Calculate the flow rate for her.

13e) Janet's feed has run for 2 hours. It then had to be stopped for 30 minutes while she went for a scan. There is 1250ml left of the feed, which should be administered over 10 hours now. Calculate the flow rate for her.

Answers are given at the end of this chapter.

Calculations: Fluid balance

An important risk assessment as part of your role and in line with NMC standards (NMC, 2018a) is to record and monitor fluid intake and output in order to identify signs of dehydration or fluid retention. Although numeracy skills involved in fluid balance are quite straightforward, the implications of incorrect calculations can significantly impact on patient safety. As well as oxygen, IV fluid and enteral feeds are prescribed medication and must be considered with the same care and safety measures as any other medication. It is imperative that the body maintains homoeostatic balance of fluid intake and loss, which is on average around 2500ml in and out per day to function properly. A loss of 2% of fluid volume is enough to trigger dehydration (Tortora and Derrickson, 2018). The core principle of fluid balance is that the amount of water lost from the body must equal the amount of water taken in. Accurate assessment of fluid balance requires adding together the total intake and output of fluids a patient has consumed via any route with the total output subtracted from the total input to obtain current fluid balance. If the output exceeds the input, this is a negative balance. This may mean that the patient is under-hydrated or dehydrated. A positive balance occurs when the input exceeds the output, which can indicate over-hydration or fluid retention. Many conditions and medications affect the intake and output of fluid which must be considered when completing fluid balance charts. Consider the impact on hydration if a patient has swallowing difficulties, cognitive impairment or peripheral oedema, or on those undergoing diuretic therapy or taking laxatives. Input and output must be considered in combination with a full assessment and observation of a patient, including vital signs, blood tests and physical observations to inform clinical decision-making. An individualised approach is needed that considers the patient, their condition and needs. Any changes or concerns with fluid balance must be escalated to a senior member of the team in accordance with Trust protocols. See Table 5.7 as an example.

Table 5.7   An example of a reasonably balanced fluid intake and output

Hours	Input				Output			
	Oral intake	IV fluids/ medication	Enteral feed	Other	Urine	Stool	Vomit	Other
01.00								
02.00					40ml			
03.00								
04.00								
05.00								
06.00					100ml			
07.00								
08.00	Sip of tea*				70ml	200ml		80ml Drain emptied
09.00		125ml			35ml			
10.00		125ml			40ml			
11.00		125ml			60ml			50ml Drain emptied
12.00		125ml	83ml		30ml			
13.00		125ml	83ml		50ml			
14.00		125ml	83ml		80ml			65ml Drain emptied
15.00		125ml	83ml					
16.00	Sip of tea*	125ml	83ml				120ml	
17.00			83ml		130ml			50ml Drain emptied
18.00			83ml					
19.00			83ml		150ml	250ml		
20.00			83ml					25ml Drain emptied
21.00			83ml		75ml			

Hours	Input				Output			
	Oral intake	IV fluids/ medication	Enteral feed	Other	Urine	Stool	Vomit	Other
22.00			83ml					
23.00	Sip of tea*		83ml		150ml			
00.00								
Total		1000ml	1000ml		1100ml	450ml	120ml	270ml
Total	2100ml				1940m l			
Fluid balance over 24hrs	+ive balance 160ml							

Note: Sips cannot be measured, so this is meaningless. Measures must be numerical values to be calculated accurately.

Table 5.7 is an example of a reasonably balanced fluid intake and output. Infusion rates (ml/hour) have been inputted hourly for accuracy. The fluid balance chart indicates that urine output was poor during the early hours of the morning, but made up for this after the IV fluids were administered. Urine output should be < 0.5ml/kg/hour to avoid kidney damage (Acute Kidney Injury), output below this therefore needs to be responded to urgently (NICE, 2019e).

If the patient is 60kg, they would need a **minimum** of 30ml per hour.

0.5 × weight (kg) = ml per hour required

0.5 × 60 = minimum of **30ml per hour**

Complete the following questions in relation to the fluid balance chart for Barry Jones who is 75kg.

Activity 5.15   Calculation practice 14

Table 5.8   Chart for calculation practice

Date:									
					Output				
Hours	Oral intake	IV fluids	IV other	Enteral feed	Other	Urine	Stool	Vomit	Other
01.00									
02.00									
03.00									
04.00									

(Continued)

Table 5.8 (Continued)

Date:

					Output				
Hours	**Oral intake**	**IV fluids**	**IV other**	**Enteral feed**	**Other**	**Urine**	**Stool**	**Vomit**	**Other**
							140ml stoma emptied		
05.00									
06.00			200ml IV antibiotics			80ml			
07.00							230ml stoma emptied	60ml	
08.00	100ml							75ml	
09.00						30ml			
10.00									
11.00						80ml			
12.00						80ml			
13.00	150ml		200ml IV antibiotics				195ml stoma emptied		
14.00						50ml		80ml	
15.00		167ml							
16.00	100ml	167ml				75ml			
17.00		167ml					120ml stoma emptied		
18.00		167ml							
19.00	80ml	167ml				100ml			
20.00		167ml							
21.00									
22.00			200ml IV antibiotics					60ml	
23.00						105ml			
00.00									
Total	?	?	?			?	?	?	
Total	?				?				

Date:

Hours	Oral intake	IV fluids	IV other	Enteral feed	Other	Urine	Stool	Vomit	Other
				Output					
Fluid balance over 24hrs	?								

14a) Calculate Barry's total daily input.

14b) Calculate Barry's total output.

14c) Is Barry in a positive or negative balance?

14d) What is the recommended urine output for Barry in light of his weight?

14e) Has Barry's urine output been adequate today?

14f) Are there any other nursing considerations that this fluid balance brings to light considering the patient's individual needs?

Answers are given at the end of this chapter.

This chapter has asked you to explore several considerations in relation to drug calculations and numeracy skills for medicines management. Activity 5.2 asked you to reflect on what you have read within the bigger picture of safe medicines management. To reflect on the factors that may influence competence in this area, let us consider Lucy's case study again.

Activity 5.16   Reflection

- What factors may have impacted on the nursing associate caring for Lucy and their ability to safely calculate medication?
- Draw on your own experiences and what you have observed in practice. How can these factors be minimised?
- Write a brief plan outlining how you hope to avoid preventable medication errors when you become qualified.

As this answer is based on your own observation and reflection, there is no outline answer at the end of this chapter.

You may wish to discuss this reflection with colleagues and retain the information in a personal portfolio.

As identified at the start of the chapter, drug calculations and numeracy skills must be retained throughout your career, so it is important that you reflect on this aspect of your clinical practice regularly in order to improve.

Now you have completed the chapter and have familiarised yourself with the numeracy skills required as part of your role, go back to Table 5.1 and consider how competent you now feel in relation to each numeracy topic. Hopefully, you now feel a little more confident and prepared approaching these numeracy tasks in practice. Competence in this area will come from theoretical knowledge as well as practical experience. Take every opportunity to practise drug calculations during placements, under appropriate supervision, to increase your confidence in these skills. Take a hard copy of the numeracy formulas displayed at the end of the Chapter 7 with you when you are in practice so you can integrate numeracy theory and practise safely. Chapter 7 will also allow you to draw on the principles discussed here, providing a range of clinical case studies to enable you to practise your numeracy skills with scenarios that relate to your clinical role and to demonstrate understanding of all the principles of safe medicines management.

Now that you have had a chance to reflect on the contents of this chapter, you can see from the following summary that you have, in fact, explored a large amount of theory and been able to link this to your own practice.

Chapter summary

This chapter has outlined the key mathematical principles needed to accurately calculate medication. Formulas have been identified to reduce medication errors and ensure safe practice in relation to this skill. The chapter has also discussed wider care-related numeracy proficiencies that are required as part of the nursing associate role, including a range of risk assessments. The importance of a systematic, logical approach to numeracy has been emphasised to reduce medication errors, as well as the importance of double-checking calculations. Professional duties and processes for reporting drug errors have also been acknowledged to prevent further harm to patients and avoid errors in the future.

Activities: Brief outline answers

Activity 5.2   Calculation practice 1 (page 81)

1a) $0.005 \times 1000 = 5$

1b) $94773 \div 1000 = 94.773$

1c) $0.8888 \times 1000 = 888.8$

1d) $94.773 \times 1000 = 94773$

1e) $111 \div 1000 = 0.111$

Activity 5.3   Calculation practice 2 (page 81)

2a)   Convert 3750mcg to grams.
      $3750 \div 1000 = 3.750g$

2b)   A patient is prescribed Naproxen 1.25g. What is this in mg?
      $1.25 \times 1000 = 1250mg$

2c) What is 0.05kg in mg?

0.05 × 1000 = 50. 50 × 1000 = **50,000mg**

2d) A 1 litre bag of Nutrison ng feed is administered. What is this in ml?

1 × 1000 = **1000ml**

2e) There is 200ml left of the 1 litre Nutrison ng feed at the end of your shift. How many ml has the patient had?

1000 − 200 = **800ml**

2f) Your patient is prescribed 3.5mg, but stock is only available in micrograms. What is 3.5mg in mcg?

3.5 × 1000 = **3500mcg**

Activity 5.4   Calculation practice 3 (page 83)

5.585

3a) Write this as a whole number.

6

3b) Write this number to 1 decimal space.

5.6

3c) Write this number to 2 decimal spaces.

5.59

Activity 5.5   Calculation practice 4 (page 83)

4a) A patient is 9.5 stones. What is this to the nearest kg?

6.35 × 9.5 = 60.325 ∴ **60kg**

4b) A mum wants to know how much her baby weighs in pounds. He is 3.2kg. Give your answer to 2 decimal spaces.

2.2 × 3.2 = **7.04lb**

4c) A patient asks you how much they weigh in stones (to the nearest whole number) if they are 85kg.

85 × 0.16 = 13.6 stones ∴ **14 stones**

4d) Convert 56lb to kg. Give your answer to the nearest whole number.

0.45 × 56 = 25.2kg ∴ **25kg**

4e) What is 6 feet in metres?

0.305 × 6 = **1.83 metres**

Activity 5.6   Calculation practice 5.5 (page 86)

5a) Nathan is 6' 2" and weighs 98kg. Calculate his BMI.

1 foot = 0.305 metres

6.2 × 0.305 = 1.891 metres

∴ 1.9 metres

height² = 1.9 × 1.9 = 3.61

BMI = 98 ÷ 3.61 = 27.1468. . .

∴ BMI = 27

5b) Julie is 1.75 metres tall and weighs 66kg. Calculate her BMI.
height² = 1.75 × 1.75 = 3.0625

BMI = 66 ÷ 3.0625 = 21.551. . .

∴BMI = 22

5c) Caroline weighs 88kg and is 5′ 3″. Calculate her BMI.
5.3 × 0.305 = 1.6165 metres

height² = 1.6 × 1.6 = 2.56

BMI = 88 ÷ 2.56 = 34.375

∴BMI = 34

5d) Is Caroline categorised as obese?
Yes

5e) Nina is 1.63 metres and weighs 40kg. Calculate her BMI.
height² = 1.63 × 1.63 = 2.6569

BMI = 40 ÷ 2.7 = 14.8148. . .

∴BMI = 15

5f) According to Figure 5.2, what is Nina's BMI score?
Score 2

Activity 5.7   Calculation practice 5.6 (page 87)

6a)   27/99 3/11

6b)   6/48 1/8

6c)   24/144 2/12 1/6

6d)   80/480 2/12 1/6

6e)   125/750 1/30

Activity 5.8   Calculation practice 7 (page 88)

7a)   What is 1/8 written as a decimal?
1 ÷ 8 = 0.125

7b)   What is 0.6 written as a percentage?
0.6 × 100 = 60%

7c)   What is 35% as a fraction in its simplest form?
32/100 = 16/50 = 8/25

7d)   What is 0.45 as a percentage?
0.45 × 100 = 45%

7e) What is 85% written as a fraction?
85/100 **17/20**

Activity 5.9 Calculation practice 8 (page 89)

8a) What is 45% of 250ml?
45 ÷ 100 × 250 = **112.5ml**

8b) There is 2% clotrimazole in a 20g tube of Canesten cream. How many grams of clotrimazole are there?
2 ÷ 100 × 20 = **0.4g**

8c) If a patient normally weighs 75kg and has lost 4500g in the last week, what is their percentage of weight loss? Round to the nearest whole number.
4500g = 4.5kg. 4.5 ÷ 100 × 75 = 3.375 ∴ **3%**

8d) You are helping the ward manager with an audit. The ward currently has 50 patients, of whom 12% have an indwelling catheter; 2% have acquired an infection from their catheter. How many patients have a catheter?
12 ÷ 100 × 50 = **6 patients**

8e) How many patients have an infection?
2 ÷ 100 × 50 = **1 patient**

Activity 5.10 Calculation practice 9 (page 91)

9a) Fluticasone cream 15g has a ratio of 1:99 (steroid:aqueous cream). How many grams of steroid are there?
15÷100 = **0.15g of steroid**

9b) Chloramphenicol eye drops 10ml are in a ratio of 1:7 (antibiotic:eye drops). How many millilitres of antibiotic is there?
10 ÷ 8 = **1.25ml**

9c) How much eye-drop solution is there?
1.25 × 7 = **8.75ml**

9d) A repeat prescription is given for chloramphenicol eye drops at a ratio of 1:7 but it is in a 5ml bottle instead of a 10ml bottle. How many ml of antibiotic is there now? Round this to 1 decimal place? 5 ÷ 8 = 0.625ml, **0.6ml**

9e) Hydramol cream has a ratio of 1 in 8 (urea: cream). How many grams of urea would there be in a tub of 500g?
500 ÷ 8 (total parts) = **62.5g**

9f) E45 has 5% urea in a 500g tub. Does E45 or Hydramol contain the most urea?
5% of 500 = 5/100 × 500 = 25g of urea in E45 ∴ **Hydramol contains the most urea**

Activity 5.11   Calculation practice 10 (page 93)

10a)   Your patient is prescribed 3.75mg bisoprolol. Tablets are available as 1.25mg. How many tablets are needed?
3.75 ÷ 1.25 = **3 tablets**

10b)   Nathan is prescribed ranitidine 150mg BD. In stock are 75mg tablets. How many tablets are needed?
150 ÷ 75 = **2 tablets**

10c)   A patient is written up for 1.5mg of diazepam. There are 500mcg tablets available in stock. How many tablets need administering?
1.5mg = 1500mcg.

500 ÷ 500 = **3 tablets**

10d)   Olivia is due 150mg trazadone as an antidepressant. Tablets in stock are 37.5mg. How many tablets will she need?
150 ÷ 37.5 = **4 tablets**

10e)   Glycerol 4g is prescribed for constipation. Suppositories in stock are 2g. How many suppositories are needed?
4 ÷ 2 = **2 suppositories**

10f)   Catherine is written up for 75mg aspirin OD. Tablets in stock are 75mg. How many tablets will she need?
75 ÷ 75 = **1 tablet**

Activity 5.12   Calculation practice 11 (page 94)

11a)   100mg Zuclopenthixol depot injection is prescribed for your patient. The solution for injection is available as 50 mg per 1 ml. How much needs to be administered?
100 ÷ 50 × 1 = **2ml**

11b)   Jason is prescribed 60mg of Phenobarbital oral solution which is available as 15mg/5ml. How much needs to be given?
60 ÷ 15 × 5 = **20ml**

11c)   Your patient has been prescribed 15mg Senna. The solution is 7.5mg/5ml. How much senna needs to be administered?
15 ÷ 7.5 = 2 × 5 = **10ml**

11d)   James is due his Actrapid insulin injection. He is written up for 30 units of insulin, the stock available is 100units/ml. How much needs to be administered?
30 ÷ 100 × 1 = **0.3 units**

11e)   Pethidine is available in stock as 100mg/2ml ampoules. Your patient is prescribed 75mg IM every 4 hours. How much needs to be administered?
75 ÷ 100 × 2 = **1.5ml**

11f)   Kate is prescribed 40mg Enoxaparin Sodium SC as post-surgery prophylaxis of deep vein thrombosis. Solution is available in stock as 20mg/0.2ml. How much needs to be administered?
40 ÷ 20 × 0.2 = **0.4ml**

Activity 5.13   Calculation practice 12 (page 96)

12a) Jenna is prescribed gentamycin 3mg/kg daily in 3 divided doses. She is 45kg. This comes in 5mg/ml solution for injection. Calculate the total daily dose needed for Jenna.

$3 \times 45 = $ **135mg per day**

12b) Calculate the dose she will need if it is divided into 3 doses in a day.

$135 \div 3 = $ **45mg per dose**

12c) Calculate the volume that needs to be administered for each individual dose.

$45 \div 5 = 9 \times 1 = $ **9ml TDS**

12d) Caden is prescribed co-amoxiclav 30mg/kg every 8 hours. Stock is available in 125mg/5ml. If he weighs 15kg, what dose will he need and how many times a day?

$30 \times 15 = $ **450mg TDS**

12e) Calculate how many millilitres need to be administered for each dose.

$450 \div 125 \times 5 = $ **18ml**

12f) Calculate the total daily dose of co-amoxiclav that Caden will have in a day.

$450mg \times 3 = $ **1350mg**

Activity 5.14   Calculation practice 13 (page 98)

13a) 500ml Nutrison multifibre feed over 5 hours is written up for your patient on a PEG feed. Calculate the flow rate for the patient.

$500 \div 5 = $ **100ml/hr**

13b) The district nurse asks you to double-check the infusion rate she has calculated for a palliative care patient while you are also at the patient's home. The patient has been prescribed morphine sulphate 20mg at a concentration of 1mg/ml over 24 hours. If the total volume is 20ml, calculate the correct flow rate for the patient. Give your answer to the nearest whole number.

$50ml \div 24 = $ **2.083ml per hour: 2ml/hr**

13c) You are asked to check the drip rate for a patient who has been prescribed 1 litre of Hartmann's IV fluids over 6 hours. A regular giving set will be used. Give your answer to the nearest whole number.

$1000 \times 20 = 20,000 \div (60 \times 6) = 20,000 \div 360 = $ 55.55555

56 drips per minute

13d) Janet is due her ng feed. She is prescribed 1500ml over 12 hours. Calculate the flow rate for her.

$1500 \div 12 = $ **125ml/hr**

13e) Janet's feed has run for 2 hours. It then had to be stopped for 30 minutes while she went for a scan. There is 1250 left of the feed which should be administered over 10 hours now. Calculate the flow rate for her.

$1250 \div 10 = $ **125m/hr**

Activity 5.15 Calculation practice 14 (page 101)

14a) Calculate Barry's total daily input.
2032ml

14b) Calculate Barry's total output.
1560ml

14c) Is Barry in a positive or negative balance?
+ive balance of 472ml

14d) What is the recommended urine output for Barry in the light of his weight? 0.5ml/ kg/hour = 0.5 ml × 75 kg = **minimum of 37.5ml per hour required**

14e) Has Barry's urine output been adequate today? **No**

14f) Are there any other nursing considerations that this fluid balance brings to light? Consider the patient's needs?

Regular bowel movements and vomiting may be adding to dehydration and may affect electrolyte balance. Vomiting seems to occur after antibiotic therapy.

Further reading

The following books are recommended to practise drug calculations and revise the principles of arithmetic in more depth.

Barber, P and Robertson, D (2020) *Essentials of Pharmacology for Nurses* (4th edn). Maidenhead: Open University Press.

Chapter 3 revises basic numeracy as well as clinical drug calculations. There are also chapters that focus on specific drug groups that contain related drug calculations at the end of each chapter.

Blair, K (2011) *Medicines Management in Children's Nursing*. Exeter: Learning Matters.

This book includes examples for managing medicines in paediatrics, including drug calculations, administration and record keeping.

Boyd, C (2021) *Calculation Skills for Nurses* (2nd edn). West Sussex: Wiley Blackwell.

This book covers all the essential calculations required for nursing associates. This resource is easy to follow, includes a range of risk assessments that require numeracy and contains plenty of practice questions at the end.

Brindley, J (2017) Undertaking drug calculations for oral medicines and suppositories. *Nursing Standard*, 32(7): 56–63.

This article discusses drug calculations in relation to practice, discussing practical ways of reducing medication errors and how to maintain competencies in this area. The same author also produced a similar article for intravenous medicines and infusions.

British National Formulary (2023). BNF Online. Retrieved from: https://bnf.nice.org.uk/

This should be used when performing drug calculations in practice to ensure that doses are correct as well as containing other crucial information to administer medication safely, as identified in the other chapters of this book.

Garford, J and Philips, N (2016) *Nursing Calculations* (9th edn). China: Elsevier.

This book covers general numeracy in depth, so may be useful if you wish to practise the basics, as there are tests as part of each section.

Hutton, M (2009) *Essential Calculation Skills for Nurses, Midwives and Healthcare Practitioners*. Maidenhead: Open University Press.

General numeracy and drug calculation formulas are included in this text, as well as sections on fluid balance and preparing different infusions. There are practice questions throughout.

Rogers, C (2017) *Calculation Skills for Nursing, Midwifery & Health Care Professionals*. London: Open University Press.

This is another resource that covers the theory of drug calculations needed for practice and provides the opportunity to complete practice questions within each section.

Starkings, S and Krause, L (2021) *Passing Calculations Tests for Nursing Students* (5th edn). London: SAGE.

This book offers advice, guidance and over 400 online questions for extra revision and practice. It aims to put the calculations required for nursing into the practical contexts you may encounter.

Tiziani, A (2015) *Drug Calculations Case Studies*. Australia: Elsevier.

This text will help you put numeracy theory into practice by working through a range of clinical case scenarios that require drug calculations. This may be a useful resource once you feel confident with your general numeracy skills and ready to apply them to practical examples.

Useful websites

The following websites are useful resources to aid safe calculation of medicines.

BMI Healthy Weight Calculator: www.nhs.uk/live-well/healthy-weight/bmi-calculator/

As discussed within this chapter, it is important to know drug equations and to use mental arithmetic to formulate answers that can then be checked with calculators. This online calculator can be used to check that BMI measurements are correct.

MUST calculator: www.bapen.org.uk/screening-and-must/must-calculator

The 'Malnutrition Universal Screening Tool' ('MUST') is an important risk assessment that involves general numeracy skills. If a paper copy is not available, the calculation can be done online using this calculator.

'MUST' printable version: www.bapen.org.uk/pdfs/must/must-full.pdf

This printable version is most commonly used in practice and is referred to in this chapter.

Electronic Medicines Compendium: www.medicines.org.uk/emc

This website allows you to search for medication and provides information on dosages as well as its pharmacokinetics and pharmacodynamics.

Medicines and Healthcare products Regulatory Agency: www.mhra.gov.uk

The Medicines and Healthcare products Regulatory Agency are responsible for ensuring that medicines and medicinal products are safe to use. This website provides regular updates regarding this.

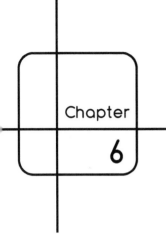

Chapter 6

Medication management in the modern age

Chapter aims

After reading this chapter, you will be able to:

- identify some of the future threats to our population's health and understand the challenges for healthcare professionals;
- identify opportunities in healthcare related to medicines optimisation and pharmacological innovations.

Introduction

Case Study: Silvi

You are shadowing a district nurse on a home visit. You visit Silvi who is 46 years old who lives with her husband and two children, Jacob who is 20 and has additional learning needs and Aida who is 6 years old. Silvi has been receiving palliative treatment for breast cancer with lymph and bone metastases. During the assessment Silvi informs you she has been having trouble sleeping. The GP has recently increased her dose of slow and immediate release morphine for regular and break through pain as her pain was not being managed effectively. She asks if there are any alternative medications or options available, she can try as she is finding some of the side effects including nausea and insomnia hard to manage.

A green paper presented to Parliament suggests that there are a number of opportunities and challenges ahead for the NHS in order to deliver health and social care in the twenty-first century (Department of Health and Social care [DHSS], 2019a). This has added meaning in the aftermath of the COVID-19 pandemic, which happened shortly after publication, the consequences of which continue to unfold globally. The consultation paper suggests that care needs to be personalised, with lifestyle advice and support targeted at the individual. Patients are no longer passive recipients of care, rather co-creators of their own health. The challenge for healthcare professionals and the government is to ensure that individuals have the skills, knowledge and confidence to achieve this.

Silvi's case study raises several issues you may encounter and an understanding of medicine management in the modern age will allow you to discuss and address some of the contemporary health concerns in your practice area. It will allow you to explore strategies for supporting your service users at all stages of life, managing their needs, promoting self-care and providing choice of both medicinal and non-pharmaceutical interventions.

Activity 6.1   Critical Thinking

Consider what some of Silvi's biopsychosocial needs are, what assessments you might utilise and what potential interventions may be needed to address her current symptoms and presenting complaints.

A short answer will be included at the end of the chapter.

As this case study demonstrates there is a need to have a clear understanding of strategies available to you to manage service users' symptoms, both physical and psychological and we will discuss these first.

Symptoms and their management

Acute pain has a protective function as the response to injury or disease. It results when tissue damage causes the stimulation of sensory, known as **nociceptive**, nerve endings found throughout the body. The initial cause of the pain, like a bee sting, results in a local release of chemicals which act on the nerve endings. In addition, **prostaglandins** are released as part of the inflammatory response. This inflammatory response includes the effects on the blood vessels resulting in tissue engorgement, the redness and swelling, and the proliferation of white cells as the immune response, known as **neurogenic inflammation**. Peripheral pain fibres run into the spinal cord and synapse with spinal cord neurons which allow for the transmission of, or stopping of, more intense pain signals to the brain. This progressing or stopping of signals describes the **gate control theory of pain** (Melzack and Wall, 1965). The brain can 'shut this gate' by the release of chemicals such as serotonin and other subjective, but less well-understood mechanisms. The sensation of pain is thought to be located in the **thalamus** and moderated by the **cerebral cortex**, but the exact physiology and function and mode of action of pain-relieving substances are still being researched.

Under normal circumstances, the sensory system returns to a normal state after healing has taken place. However, if features of sensation persist, and by definition for a period of greater than 6 months, it may manifest as chronic pain. **Chronic pain** is characterised by the abnormal state and function of the neurons in the spinal cord which become hyperactive. This is a result of increased transmitter release by neurons and an increased responsiveness of the receptors. In addition, there is the loss of function of inhibitory neurons which would usually moderate the pain. Genetic and environmental factors can contribute to this hypersensitivity leading to permanent structural changes in the area of the brain responsible for nociceptor regulation. Treatment aims to decrease the intensity of acute pain and therefore reduce or prevent the permanent changes to the nervous system which may result in chronic pain. Therapies including appropriate combinations of medications and adjuvants are used.

Palliative care, the treatment, care and support for people with life-limiting illness often involves the need to control pain as well as other distressing symptoms such as nausea, breathlessness and agitation in order to promote quality for remaining life. Regardless of the type and source of pain, the treatment aim is to alleviate or reduce the sensation of pain which requires assessment and treatment with analgesics and/or non-pharmaceutical methods. The World Health Organisation (1986) proposed the analgesic ladder – 'by the clock, by the mouth, by the ladder' as a means of ensuring timely, least invasive and sequential strength of medicated response to alleviate pain.

Within your practice environments you will encounter a number of assessment tools which will allow your service user to communicate their level of pain, these can be adapted for use with children and adults with intellectual disabilities, or those with cognitive decline and allow for an appropriate response from you.

Aspirin and paracetamol are the most common analgesics taken for pain management for adults. Their exact modes of action are unknown, but they have been found to benefit headache, muscle pains and arthritis but are ineffective for visceral pain. They have a weak non-steroidal anti-inflammatory (NSAID) effect and a number of toxic and advisory notices (BNF, 2023).

NSAIDs, like ibuprofen, are used for the management of moderate pain due to tissue inflammation. NSAIDs vary in both analgesic and anti-inflammatory potency and in the severity of side effects which they all share, including gastro-intestinal perforation and haemorrhage, acute renal failure and asthma exacerbation. As always there is the need to review the BNF before they are administered.

Morphine and diamorphine are the strongest analgesics known. Pharmaceutical companies have synthesised other less effective products, including codeine, pethidine, fentanyl, buprenorphine and others. As **opiates** these medications are thought to work in the mid-brain and cerebral cortex causing feelings of wellbeing and tranquility, known as euphoria, and allow for the closing of the pain gate by inhibiting pain receptors. The range of opiates are used for a variety of clinical situations and generally share the same range of side effects and the potential for misuse. Opiates are lethal in overdose. The drug naloxone may be used as a competitive antagonist for the opiate receptors which prevents the binding of the opiate to its receptor therefore reversing its effect.

There are a range of circumstances which may result in **nausea and vomiting** for your patient. Including as a side effect of other medication, as in the case study. Targeted care will include not only the symptom management but also investigation of the underlying cause. The most commonly prescribed include those which encourage peristalsis and speed up gastric emptying like metoclopramide and domperidone. Others include the antihistamines like cyclizine and the 5-HT3 receptor antagonists, for example, ondansetron. As with all medications notable contra-indications and cautions exist. Metoclopramide may be associated with extrapyramidal neurological symptoms, cyclizine with euphoric and psychoactive effects and ondansetron with cardiac implications. Therefore, safe administration requires the scrutiny of the BNF for specific concerns.

For abnormal bowel function, as with all patient care, the priority for treatment will include the investigation of underlying causes. For **diarrhoea**, the restoration and maintenance of hydration and electrolyte balance along with the restoration of normal bowel function is required. Rehydration treatments may include the over-the-counter product dioralyte along with the encouragement of increased oral fluid intake. **Antimotility** medications slow down bowel peristalsis (see chapter 2). They allow increased water absorption to allow for normal stool formation and can be given short term for the comfort of your patients; they include codeine phosphate and loperamide as examples. Medications to relieve **constipation** are known as **laxatives** and include bulk-forming, osmotic, stimulant and faecal softeners. Their mode of action is complex and include fybogel, movicol, lactulose, senna, glycerol and arachis oil as examples. Constipation is a commonly encountered complaint and along with investigating cause you will need to be sympathetic to your patient's perceptions of a normal bowel habit and as always review the BNF for specific concerns.

Dyspepsia, or indigestion, has a variety of causes including obesity, food intolerance, smoking, high alcohol intake and a variety of medical conditions and their treatments. It is characterised by discomfort in the upper abdomen known as heartburn. It may be associated with the symptoms of bloating, belching, nausea and anorexia. Treatments depend largely on the cause of the dyspepsia and include antacids which may be bought over the counter, such as gaviscon, which neutralises and prevents acid reflux providing relief. Further treatments include histamine antagonists which block the histamine receptors in the stomach so preventing the release of gastric acid. Proton pump inhibitors, for example, omeprazole, prevent the pumping of hydrogen ions into the stomach preventing gastric acid formation. Vigilance and close monitoring of your patients will ensure that serious gastro-intestinal pathology such as gastric cancer is not missed during symptom management of dyspepsia.

Inflammatory symptoms include several features.

- **Pyrexia** is a natural immune response which results in a high core body temperature, otherwise known as a fever, and is a mechanism aimed to reduce bacterial and viral multiplication. The hypothalamus responds to the presence of substances called **pyrogens** which are released into the circulatory system from injured tissues or from the presence of micro-organisms. Antipyretics including paracetamol and NSAIDS may be used for symptom relief, but an awareness of contraindications and interactions is required. In many circumstances, non-medication symptom relief, like tepid bathing for example, is advocated.

- Urticaria, a condition characterised by the appearance of itchy weals on the skin, is the result of a hypersensitivity reaction. Investigation to the cause is required and from a medicine management perspective an assessment and review of all recently administered medicines is required. Acute life-threatening adverse reactions require an appropriate emergency response (see Chapter 4).
- Pruritus or itching can occur. This is thought to be the result of simulation of the subepidermal nerve plexus by proteolytic enzymes that are released from the epidermis as a result of a primary irritation. It can be generalised or systemic, the result of a skin condition or a feature of a systemic disorder. Where possible the underlying cause should be treated. Emollients may assist with symptom control where the pruritis is associated with dry skin. Treatment including topical agents like hydrocortisone cream 1 per cent or betnovate-RD may be used to relieve symptoms and suppress signs of the disorder when other measures like emollients are not effective (BNF, 2023).

As well as acute physical symptoms your service users may be affected by psychological symptoms. **Affective disorders** are characterised by disturbances of mood and can be the result of anxiety, depression and conditions like dementia.

For **anxiety,** the anxiolytics and hypnotic medications may be used, although the NICE, (2019b) guideline recommends psychosocial rather than medicinal treatments. Sleep disturbances can be treated with benzodiazepines, for example, temazepam and nitrazepam, in the short term due to their high degree of tolerance and dependence. Non-benzodiazepines which function at the same receptors may also be prescribed, an example being zopiclone.

Depression can be associated with symptoms such as insomnia, altered appetite, social withdrawal and suicidal ideation. The most used antidepressants, and recommended by NICE (2019c), are the selective serotonin reuptake inhibitors (SSRIs) as generally they are associated with less side effects. They work by blocking serotonin, a neurotransmitter, from returning to the neuron, increasing its action. Monoamine oxidase inhibitors are used less frequently as they are associated with more interactions with certain foods and can affect blood pressure. Antidepressant medication usually takes at least three weeks to have an effect. The medications amitriptyline, sertraline, mirtazapine and venlafaxine are effective for many service users, although not all and approaches such as cognitive behavioural therapy in combination with medication, or on its own, are recommended to maximise the benefit of treatment (BNF, 2023).

Dementia can be associated with a wide range of symptoms including cognitive impairment, thought to be as a result of degeneration of neurons in the amygdala and can be treated with cholinesterase inhibitors including donepezil, galantamine and rivastigmine (NICE, 2018).

Acute psychotic episodes may result in distressing symptoms for your service users. Medications, sometimes described as neuroleptics, with a wide variety of structures have anti-psychotic effects. Broadly they work by blocking dopamine receptors, as a dopamine antagonist, and have varying severity in adverse effects. Individual responses remain idiosyncratic and the best treatment for an individual may be subject to trial and error. Examples include chlorpromazine, fluphenazine, haloperidol and clozapine. Community treatments often include long-acting oily depot injections for maintenance therapy which may increase the incidence of movement disorders. Treatment adherence is a major clinical issue, however, impacting on areas such as safety, relapse and long-term prognosis. The effectiveness and side effects have a major impact on concordance.

Having explored common symptom management with medicine administration, it is important to remind ourselves that non-pharmaceutical options and alternative therapies may be used.

Complementary and alternative medicines

Complementary and alternative medicines (CAMs) refer to a diverse group of therapies and disciplines that are not considered part of mainstream healthcare. They include health-related therapies which have roots in historical, cultural or religious practices; their philosophies being fundamentally holistic and individualistic.

There has been a significant increase in the use of CAMs in recent years. This rise in popularity may have been influenced by a rise in consumer knowledge and people becoming disenchanted with dominant healthcare treatments. These therapies have been classified by the House of Lords (2000) into three broad categories. Within these classifications, some CAMs have well-developed regulatory structures and have begun to build an evidence base while others are fragmented practitioners with little agreement about regulation (See Table 6.1).

Table 6.1   House of Lords Select Committee on Science and Technology report (2000)

Group	Description	Examples
1	Most established form of CAM that have diagnostic method and are most advanced in terms of regulated practice. Have greatest evidence for efficacy – often referred to as 'big five' therapies.	Osteopathy, chiropractic, acupuncture, herbal medicine and homeopathy
2	Normally used to compliment conventional medicine. Do not claim to make diagnosis.	Aromatherapy, alexander technique, massage, counselling, stress therapy, hypnotherapy, reflexology, shiatsu and meditation
3a	Offer therapeutic as well as diagnostic service. Involve a philosophy which does not relate to conventional medicine – 2 subgroups	a) Traditional Chinese and Ayurvedic medicine
3b	Number of disciplines which lack evidence base	b) Crystal therapy, dowsing and kinesiology, iridology and radionics

As a nursing associate you need to be aware of the debate surrounding benefits and pitfalls of CAMs and the contraindications and conflicts between them and mainstream healthcare. Many of your patients will be accessing these therapies for either an acute condition or end of life prognosis and you will have a responsibility to support your service users to access reliable evidence to allow them to make informed choices about their care. Since a variety of therapies and disciplines exist, you are encouraged to access appropriate literature on specific CAMs if accessing them yourself or for your patients, relying on good quality evidence to inform your practice. In the case study at the beginning of this chapter you would need to assist Silvi to access evidence-based information to enable an informed decision on whether reflexology or aromatherapy could aid her in her insomnia for example.

Complementary and alternative medicines are often accessed by service users to alleviate both acute and chronic symptoms of discomfort and regardless of efficacy are seen to have a psychological impact, giving people hope for the alleviation of their symptoms. This beneficial effect which cannot be attributed to the medicinal or therapy properties is described as the placebo effect. It is a result of the patient's belief in that treatment. Placebo effects can be attributed to both CAMs and conventional medical therapies.

Social prescribing

Non-pharmacological treatment can be utilised with referral to 'activities' or services in the community instead of offering only medical solutions. Social prescribing is being recognised as a way of reducing polypharmacy (DHSS, 2019a; RPS, 2013) and can complement or replace pharmacological treatments. It enables GPs, nurses and other health and care professionals to refer people to a range of local, non-clinical services as a key component of universal personalised care. If Silvi requires more support, she may benefit from a social prescribing link worker who could develop a personalised care plan to promote her wellbeing and that of her family. This could include physical activity and rehabilitation prescriptions to promote quality of life.

As access to CAMs and social prescribing is often for symptom management, activity 6.1 asks you to reflect on your current knowledge of commonly encountered symptoms.

Activity 6.2   Reflection

Think of examples of symptoms you have had reported in practice. What pharmaceutical, social or innovative prescribing therapies have you observed being used to alleviate distress.

As this answer is based on your own observation and reflection, there is no outline answer at the end of this chapter.

You may wish to discuss this reflection with colleagues and retain the information in a personal portfolio.

Challenges for healthcare

Having explored strategies for symptom management, we are now going to review some of the challenges healthcare professionals face in modern medicines management.

Antimicrobial resistance

Antimicrobial resistance (AMR) is a worldwide challenge which requires a global response to antibiotic stewardship. AMR occurs when microorganisms such as bacteria, viruses, fungi and parasites adapt and mutate in ways that render medications used to cure the infections they cause ineffective (WHO, 2017a). AMR occurs naturally, through the transfer of genetic material, but is facilitated by the inappropriate use of antibacterial medicines, for example, the use of antibiotics to attempt to treat viral infections and the overuse of broad-spectrum antibiotics. **Antimicrobial stewardship** is therefore required and is defined as, 'an organisa-tional or healthcare-system-wide approach to promoting and monitoring judicious use of antimicrobials to preserve their future effectiveness' (NICE, 2015a, p2).

Before selecting an antibacterial, the prescriber must consider both the individual and the likely causative organism. Local policies often limit the antibacterial that may be used to achieve reasonable economy consistent with adequate cover and to reduce the development of resistant organisms (BNF, 2023).

NICE (2019d) antimicrobial prescribing guidelines have been developed to promote pru-dent prescribing of antibiotics as well as justifying whether antibiotics are needed to support a clinician's decision-making. Shorter courses of treatment are also recommended to reduce resistance. This is also likely to increase concordance.

The use of broad-spectrum antibiotics is discouraged for antibiotic stewardship and for clinical reasons; there is evidence that their use is associated with increased rates of clos-tridium difficile (NICE, 2015b). This is because the antibiotic action of killing or preventing bacteria from replicating will influence the normal, healthy gut microbiome (see Chapter 2) and allow for the infiltration of pathogenic bacteria. This is the reason why gastric side effects are often associated with antibiotic use.

There are occasions when broad spectrum antibiotics are indicated, however. In the case of sepsis, broad-spectrum antibiotics are necessary to treat a wide range of possible microor-ganisms that may be causing the systemic infection (Nutbeam & Daniels on behalf of UK Sepsis Trust, 2019). Sepsis is defined as the association of non-specific inflammatory responses with evidence, or suspicion, of a microbial origin. When accompanied by evidence of reduced perfusion or dysfunction of at least one organ system, this becomes severe sepsis. Where severe sepsis is accompanied by hypotension or need for vasopressors, despite adequate fluid resuscitation, the term septic shock applies (Nutbeam & Daniels on behalf of UK, Sepsis, 2019). Increasing severity correlates with increasing mortality.

Worldwide sepsis affects 48.9 million people with 11 million deaths accounting for 20 per cent of all global deaths. In 2017, almost half of these cases were among children with 2.9 million deaths in children under five years of age (WHO, 2020). Thus, sepsis is a medical emergency. Awareness and recognition are key and as a nursing associate you will need to be aware of the sepsis pathways and treatment regimes in your area of practice. The urgency of treatment of adult and paediatric patients with suspected sepsis is based on National Early Warning Scores in secondary care (NEWS2 for adults, PEWS for children) combined with clinical and laboratory assessments of severity, urgency and probability of infection – see NICE guideline NG 51 (2022). The treatment framework allows sufficient time to make an informed clinical judgement with antimicrobial treatment being accompanied by source identification, control and antimicrobial stewardship (Academy of Medical Colleges, 2022)

Before proceeding it would be a good idea to familiarise yourself with your own organi-sations' policies and procedures in the event of caring for an individual with sepsis, and activity 6.3 invites you to do this.

Activity 6.3 Work-based learning

Review your organisations' policies and procedures for identifying and responding to service users with sepsis.

This answer is based on your own observation; there is however an answer outlining the 'sepsis six' at the end of this chapter.

Now that you have reviewed your organisations' polices for identifying and treating those individuals with sepsis, let us continue to explore the challenges associated with antibiotic administration.

In January 2019, the UK Government published a 20-year vision and 5-year national action plan for how the UK will contribute to containing and controlling AMR. This is to ensure current antibiotics stay effective, reduce the numbers of resistant infections, support appropriate prescribing practices and to encourage the pharmaceutical industry to take more responsibility (DHSS, 2019b). In 2022, WHO additionally stated its intention to continue collaborative strategies for AMR alongside preparedness for pandemic initiatives.

As trainees and registrants, you will have a responsibility to educate service users about when antibiotics are needed and how to ensure correct use. You will have a role and responsibility to promote infection control and reduce hospital and healthcare acquired infections as an **antibiotic guardian.** You will also need to understand your role in identifying and responding to service users with the life-threatening condition of sepsis.

Immunisation and public perception

Vaccination against disease is one of the most cost-effective interventions in healthcare. It protects the general population, and through herd immunity, allows for the protection of vulnerable groups. Herd immunity describes how a population is protected from a disease after vaccination by stopping the microorganism responsible for the infection being transmitted between people. In this way, individuals who cannot be vaccinated can be protected. Many parents are reluctant to have their children immunised against childhood diseases for fear of side effects of the immunisation itself, however. This followed a widely publicised 1998 study by a UK Dr Wakefield who suggested that the MMR vaccine might cause autism. This claim has since been retracted by his co-authors, but immunisation rates are still to recover fully and this was not before outbreaks had resulted in thousands of cases of measles, hundreds of hospitalisations and at least three deaths (Quick and Larson, 2018).

Vaccine hesitancy has been identified within the WHO's (WHO, 2019) 5-year strategic plan as one of the 10 issues that will demand attention from WHO and health partners. They suggest that the reluctance or refusal to vaccinate against vaccine-preventable diseases while being a complex issue is largely a result of complacency, inconvenience in accessing vaccines and lack of confidence. This was demonstrated clearly with the recent COVID-19 pandemic and re-iterates the importance of drawing on evidence base for your practice.

Activity 6.4   Reflection

Consider how you would approach a vulnerable patient who has been influenced by media accounts and is declining routine vaccinations.

As the answers are based on your own observation and reflection, there are no outline answers at the end of this chapter. You may wish to discuss this reflection with colleagues and retain the information in a personal portfolio.

Potential for drug misuse

Drug dependence occurs when the body's systems adapt to the repeated exposure to a medicine and only functions normally in the presence of that medicine. When the drug is withdrawn, several reactions occur, these can be physical and psychological. Known as the withdrawal syndrome, the reactions vary from the mild to life threatening. The individual may take the substance again to avoid the physiological and psychological distress associated with the withdrawal syndrome. A variety of substances may incur a dependence, from caffeine in food and drink, nicotine in cigarettes, analgesics taken to relieve acute pain, like opioid medication, and sedatives taken to aid sleep. There is also the potential for abuse of non-dependence-producing substances (WHO, 2018b). This is defined as repeated and inappropriate use of a substance which, though the substance has no dependence potential, is accompanied by harmful or psychological effects, or involves unnecessary contact with health professionals. A variety of medicines may be involved, including over-the-counter medicines, prescribed and herbal remedies. These substances while they do not have the potential for dependence in the sense of their pharmaceutical effects, they can produce a psychological dependence.

Drug misuse is defined as the use of a substance for a purpose not consistent with legal or medical guidelines (WHO, 2018b). It is associated with a range of harms including poor physical and mental health and sociological effects such as relationship breakdown unemployment and homelessness and therefore has a negative impact on health and functioning. It may take the form of drug dependence or be part of a wider spectrum of problematic or harmful behaviour.

When considering the case study, however, in palliative care, pain and symptom control should be your primary concern and not the dependence of substances as your aim is to alleviate pain and distress in terminal illness.

Changing political agenda

A further challenge is the impact politics has on medicines management. Under Brexit, the United Kingdom entered a new era for the pharmaceutical industry. The UK Trade and Cooperation Agreement with the EU came into effect in 2021. This attempts to ensure smooth trade between EU and the UK as jurisdiction and legal obligations have separated. The MHRA now independently regulates for England, Scotland and Wales. At the time of writing, there are still a number of challenges and concerns for the industry to address. Throughout your career as a nursing associate, you will be influenced by the political agenda of the time for all aspects of healthcare, including medicines management and an awareness and understanding of implications for you and your service users will be essential to help you fulfill your role.

Global threats to health

A final consideration is the global challenge associated with epidemics, pandemics and the required international response. The COVID-19 pandemic is a recent example of this. The race to identify effective treatments to combat threats is challenging but allows for opportunities and innovations in public health provision and medicines management.

Opportunities for healthcare

New medicine development

A major opportunity for the future of disease and symptom control is the development of new medicines to prevent, treat or reduce severity of illnesses. The starting point for this is research into disease processes at a molecular and cellular level. Through better understanding of disease development, a specific gene or protein instrumental to the progression of the disease may be identified which a new medicinal product could have an effect on. An example of this would be the development of a product that blocks an essential receptor. Historically this search would have been among natural substances in plants and animals, but in modern times synthetic substances are often computer generated and formulated. The start of a long and detailed trial and testing process is then required. Product safety and efficacy tests are conducted using computerised models, simulation and preclinical trials. Many new products do not make it past this initial testing phase. In the UK, approval for the next stage of clinical trial is required from the Medicines and Healthcare products Regulatory agency (MHRA). If they consider that enough preliminary research has been conducted, they will allow closely controlled testing on healthy volunteers. Many products do not make it through this stage either, because they turn out to be ineffective, have safety concerns or unacceptable side effects. Those that do get through can be trialled on a larger section of the population. In England and Wales, these new products need to be recommended by the National Institute of Health and Care Excellence (NICE) to allow prescribers to have access to them on the NHS. The decision to allow access depends on the determined benefit to the general population. Prescribing guidelines are then based on the best available evidence to ensure safe and effective care. This is known as clinical effectiveness and once this is established, cost effectiveness is considered. Finally, many countries, including the UK, will require pharmacovigilance, the surveillance of the new products, to monitor the medicine once it is in general use (see Chapter 4).

As well as new medications, trials can be undertaken with current licensed medications to discover new benefits. During the pandemic, research such as the Recovery trial tested a range of already licensed medications for the treatment of COVID-19. Certain drugs such as dexamethasone were found to reduce deaths by 30 per cent in patients with severe illness (Recovery, 2020). This treatment has now been embedded in NICE clinical guidelines for treating COVID-19 (NICE, 2022).

Innovative medicine delivery and diagnostic systems

As well as new medicines, innovative approaches to treatment delivery mechanisms are being investigated. For example, the Massachusetts Institute of Technology (MIT) have developed a pill coated with many tiny needles that could be used to inject medicines like insulin and antibiotics into the lining of the stomach or small intestine. They are also researching the possibility of electronic pills which can release drugs in response to smart phone commands (MIT, 2021). Additionally, a clinical trial has been exploring whether the Cytosponge TFF3, a sponge on a string pill test can help detect early signs of Barrett's oesophageal cancer. Results have shown that this quick and easy to use pill can detect 10 times the amount of abnormalities in comparison to treatment as usual (NIHR, 2022). These experimental but innovative means of aiding diagnosis and delivering medicines to service users with long-term conditions offer a range of opportunities for better medicine management and optimisation. They are aligned to the WHO's commitment to virtual interventions, the increase of self-care and self-testing innovations (WHO, 2022).

Genomics

It has been known for some time that genetic factors play a role in our individual health. The human genome, our DNA within our 23 chromosome pairs, defines how we develop, maintain homeostasis and ultimately defines our differences from one another. By investigating and sequencing DNA, known as the science of **genomics**, it is possible to identify individuals at risk from specific disease processes. Early diagnosis in this way allows individuals to make lifestyle changes which may prevent disease or lessen its impact, lead to more effective prescription medicines and focussed health interventions. Statins, also known as HMG-CoA reductase inhibitors, as an example, could lower serum lipids and reduce illness and mortality in those who are at risk of cardiovascular disease. This is a further WHO (2022) innovation commitment. They have advocated a range of tools and funding processes to make genomic technology more affordable for less-resourced countries so that all may benefit.

Artificial intelligence

The NHS Long Term Plan outlined its vision for the future of the NHS, drawing on innovations in technology to enhance all aspects of service provision (NHS England, 2019b). A National Artificial Intelligence lab was created to look at ways of using technology to improve healthcare through enhancing screening processes, developing algorithms to improve patient safety and using digital tools to assist with diagnosis and treatment. In 2022, the WHO and the International Digital Health and AI Research Collaborative (I-DAIR) have signed a memorandum of understanding outlining their joint efforts to advance the use of digital technologies globally.

The use of smart devices for health benefits is a growing phenomenon. Artificial intelligence (AI) allows healthcare professions to create models of care from anonymised clinical data obtained from smart devices worn by service users to inform treatment regimens. Public Health England (PHE) and the NHS have through the UK Biobank, been able to build a record of data from volunteers to plan both targeted public health messages and to begin to inform policy (DHSS, 2019a). There are challenges that will need to be overcome to optimise these innovations. This includes developing the current technological infrastructure to enable digital capabilities, such as having integrated digital care records across all settings as well as ensuring new technology complies with data protection and privacy regulations (see Chapter 1).

Amongst the innovations within this area is the potential to use these strategies to promote self-management and healthy lifestyles.

Supporting healthy lifestyle choices

As a nursing associate you will be aware of the impact lifestyle has on your patients' health. With both the choices service users make and the environmental and economic factors affecting their health and wellbeing. Poor lifestyle choices and circumstances represent one of the largest challenges to health in developed countries and we will briefly explore some of the main opportunities for intervention next.

Smoking cessation

Smoking has a well-known impact on the respiratory and other body systems. Nicotine dependence is the most common drug dependence in the UK and the biggest cause of avoidable premature deaths (DHSS, 2019a). The use of health promotion education and supportive cessation products, including medications like nicotine replacement patches are essential to assist smokers to quit. Additionally, e-cigarettes, as an alternative, are being assessed as a way to deliver nicotine as a safer alternative to tobacco smoking (Independent Committee on Toxicity, 2017; PHE, 2019). There are also claims that heated tobacco products could be less harmful than smoking and help smokers quit. The DH (2019a) still recommend that smokers quit rather than moving onto e-cigarette or heated tobacco products.

Maintaining a healthy weight

Obesity, as a result of poor lifestyle choices is well recognised as a challenge for current and future healthcare services. Only a third of adults in UK are a healthy weight with 1 in 3 children aged 10–11 overweight. Obese children we know are 5 times more likely to become obese adults (DHSS, 2019a) and this reduces life expectancy by average of 9 years (PHE, 2017).

Medication can be used in combination with lifestyle advice. In 2023, NICE recommended a weight-loss drug be made available in specialist NHS services (TA875). This once-a-week injection from a pre-filled syringe containing semaglutide has been shown to suppresses appetite (NICE, 2023).

Social prescribing

As a non-pharmacological treatment, social prescribing can be utilised with referral to 'activities' or services in the community instead of offering only medical solutions. Social prescribing is being recognised as a way of reducing polypharmacy (DHSS, 2019a; RPS, 2013) and can complement or replace pharmacological treatments. Otherwise it is acknowledged that the NHS will continue to be treating the symptoms of problems rather than addressing the causes.

Reducing alcohol consumption

High alcohol consumption has a known impact on physical health and associated psychological and sociological effects (DHSS, 2019a). Abstinence with supportive counselling can be helped by medication, such as disulfiram, which inhibits removal of alcohol metabolites inducing the unpleasant effects of sweating, nausea and vomiting. Replacement of thiamine (vitamin B1) may be required additionally as alcohol inhibits its uptake from the GI tract. Benzodiazepines maybe required to prevent seizure associated with alcohol withdrawal.

Maintaining mental health

Additionally, one of the developing challenges for modern healthcare is the recognition that mental health must be given equal priority to physical health (NHS England, 2018). This 'Parity of esteem' was enshrined in UK law in 2012 and demands equal access, availability and resources for both physical and mental health services. Social prescribing is one way in which services are addressing this.

Addressing inequality of health outcomes

There are a number of service user groups who have poorer outcomes when engaging with services and this has been identified as a key challenge for modern healthcare globally.

Refugees and migrants

Displacement is known to be a key factor in health and wellbeing and poorer health outcomes are apparent in migrant and refugee populations (WHO, 2022).

Gender

Gender norms, roles and relations impact on health-related behaviours and outcomes. Appropriate health sector responses are key. The Global action for Trans Equality (GATE) recognises the vulnerability of marginalised individuals to Human Immunological Virus (HIV), viral hepatitis and sexually transmitted diseases (WHO, 2022). Global health strategies are required to ensure equality of access to diagnosis and treatments.

Learning disability

Individuals who are unable to communicate effectively are at greater risk of poor health service outcomes. As a nursing associate you have a moral, ethical and professional obligation to advocate for all individuals (NMC, 2018b). A number of tools and resources are available to assist in assessment of specific issues. People with learning disability are four times more likely to be suffering from a mental illness, for example, and require tailored medication responses. They are also prone to syndromes associated with difficult to control seizures (Gates et al., 2015).

Consider for a moment, Jacob in the case study, he may not fully understand the implications of his mother's illness and may need additional support around this time. An advanced care plan can include the needs of family members as well as documentation of conversations around end-of-life planning, preferences and wishes.

Understanding the theory: Medicine management in the modern age

While the complete understanding of the challenges and opportunities for healthcare may seem complex when you first consider it, it will be something you have been aware of already in your daily practice. You have cared for service users in line with up-to-date organisation's policies. You will have discussed the political agenda and new healthcare discoveries and been aware of recent changes in healthcare provision. In addition, you will be familiar with the general feelings towards health and healthcare within the population, printed and social media. All of these will have acknowledged some of the current challenges and opportunities within healthcare and medicine management. We all encounter these opportunities and threats within our daily practice which will evolve over time as will our responses to them. The use of evidence-based organisational policies and having an awareness of healthcare-related media coverage and the current political agenda and how these impact on healthcare provision allow us to deliver the highest standards of care. Anyone working within modern healthcare is familiar with change, its impact on the service user and the need to keep up to date. This is an example of you putting the theory into practice.

Now that you have explored and recognised some of the challenges and opportunities within modern healthcare, take some time to reflect on what you have learnt which will additionally allow you to apply to it your practice. Activity 6.5 will help you with this.

Activity 6.5   Critical thinking

1. List some of the opportunities available for improved medicines management.

2. Explain your role in assisting service users to choose pharmaceutical and non-pharmaceutical therapies for symptom management.

3. Give some examples of lifestyle choices which may affect health and medicines management.

4. How do you define sepsis and how would you respond as a nursing associate?

5. Write down at least 3 ways you can be an antibiotic guardian within your everyday practice.

There are no sample answers to these questions.

Where you are not confident in your knowledge of a topic, you may find it necessary to re-read sections of this chapter or view the further reading and websites listed at the end of this chapter to assist you. Information for Question 1 can be found in the first section of this chapter. Question 2 in the complementary and alternative therapies section, question 3 in the lifestyle and implications for health table, question 4 and 5 in the last section of this chapter exploring some of the challenges for modern healthcare.

Chapter summary

You have discovered from this chapter that medicine management in the modern age needs to address some of the contemporary health concerns and threats to our population's health and embrace the opportunities for innovation in healthcare. This chapter has outlined some of those opportunities including new medicine development, the use of technology, AI and precision medicine. This chapter has outlined complementary therapies and has discussed some of the commonly encountered symptoms for your service users. In addition, the challenges associated with antibiotic resistance and stewardship have been explored and sepsis defined. Other challenges including immunisation hesitancy, drug misuse and the effect of poor lifestyle choices have been examined. Finally, the need to be aware of the current political agenda has been highlighted. The activities within this chapter asked you to reflect on your knowledge of commonly encountered symptoms and to consider the medicinal, alternative and innovative therapies to alleviate distress which you have observed in use. In addition to demonstrate your understanding of sepsis and your role in recognising and treating this life-threatening condition.

Activities brief outline answers

Activity 6.1: Critical thinking

Consider what some of Silvi's biopsychosocial needs are, what assessments can you utilise and what potentials interventions may be needed to address her current symptoms and presenting complaints?

- A range of pain assessments – analgesics, non-pharmacological pain interventions such as CAMs, social prescribing
- Assessment of nausea and vomiting – antiemetics, peppermint water, CAMs
- Medication review
- Vital signs
- Mental health assessment – antidepressants, talking therapies or a combination
- Social support including the children and how they are coping – social prescribing
- Consideration of financial implications – social prescribing
- Mobility assessment – mobility aids, rehabilitation, physiotherapy, CAMs, social prescribing
- Nutritional status – supplements
- Conversations around end-of-life (EOL) care decisions, legalities including DNAR and power of attorney and documenting wishes and preferences in EOL
- Silvi and her family need a holistic assessment of their needs, including consideration of wider social, financial, cultural and psychological factors (GSF, 2022). Advanced care planning is one way of enabling personalised care that is tailored to the individual, enabling them to have control and choice over their own care.

Now that you have had a chance to reflect on how opportunities and challenges impact you in practice, you can see from the following summary that you have in fact explored a large amount of theory and been able to link this to your own practice.

Further reading

The following books are recommended for this chapter.

Ashelford, S, Raynsford, J and Taylor, V (2024) *Pathophysiology and Pharmacology for Nursing Students* (3rd edn). London: SAGE.

This textbook introduces the core concepts of key pathophysiological processes useful for the further understanding of symptom management. Chapter 2 explains the way the body responds to injury and infection; Chapter 3 informs the reader of the main infectious micro-organisms; Chapters 6 and 7 focus on pain and nausea, and vomiting mechanisms.

Levy, M, Evans, L and Rhodes, A (2018) The Surviving Sepsis campaign bundle: 2018 update. *Intensive Care Medicine*, 44(6): 925–8.

This article explores the evidence behind the Sepsis Six bundle and explains the rationale behind the assessments, treatment and necessity of a timely response when sepsis is suspected.

Neal, MJ (2020) *Medical Pharmacology at a Glance* (9th edn). Chichester: Wiley Blackwell.

This illustrated text written for medical students offers a concise introduction to medicines pharmacology and includes examples of commonly prescribed treatments with mechanisms of action and cautionary advice.

Spires, A and O'Brien, M (2011) *Introduction to Medicines Management in Nursing.* Exeter: Learning Matters.

Chapter 4 offers alternative approaches to medicines in nursing and describes the history of CAMs, an overview of some regularly encountered techniques, as well as explores factors that affect patient choice. Chapter 6 examines medicines management in field-specific care environments and is useful to further explore symptom management.

Useful websites

The following websites are resources to aid your understanding.

BNF Publications: www.bnf.org

This website allows you to search for specific medicine information and guides for symptom management.

National Institute for Health and Clinical Excellence: www.nice.org.uk

The NICE (2019b) guidance includes information on treatment options for service users with anxiety and depression, NICE (2018) guidance on dementia care and NICE (2018) the impact of antimicrobial resistance.

Specialist Pharmacy Service: www.sps.nhs.uk/

This website offers professional medicines advice, including antimicrobial resistance networks.

The UK Sepsis Trust: https://sepsistrust.org/https://sepsistrust.org/wp-content/uploads/2020/01/Sepsis-Acute-12-1.3.pdf

The UK Sepsis Trust exists as a resource to stop preventable deaths and support those affected. Includes guidance treatment pathways for in-patient and community settings. The Sepsis Trust has recently updated their screening tool and clinical guidance, which is a very useful resource for both trainee nursing associates and qualified staff to ensure safe and timely care for patients with suspected sepsis.

Antibiotic Guardian: https://antibioticguardian.com/

This is a Public Health England campaign that started in 2014 to raise awareness about the growing public health problem of antibiotic resistance. There are quizzes and crosswords to test your knowledge in this area as well as leaflets for healthcare professionals and the general public on how to tackle this global issue.

Health Matters: Antimicrobial resistance (Public Health England, 2015): www.gov.uk/government/publications/health-matters-antimicrobial-resistance/health-matters-antimicrobial-resistance

Health Matters: Antimicrobial resistance (Public Health England, 2015) provides an overview of this growing problem and how we all have a role in reducing antimicrobial resistance. This document signposts to other useful resources and where to get further information.

Royal College of Nursing: www.rcn.org.uk/clinical-topics/public-health/self-care/social-prescribing

A Royal College of Nursing resource explaining what social prescribing is, how it works and examples of where it is making a positive impact on communities.

Healthy Homes. Accommodating an Ageing Population: http://allcatsrgrey.org.uk/wp/download/housing/imeche-healthy-homes-report.pdf?platform=hootsuite

An interesting read about the use of artificial intelligence in our service users' homes to assist with monitoring safety, and to optimise health and maintain independence, particularly in the older population.

Genomics England: https://www.genomicsengland.co.uk/

A UK genomics database that is gathering genomic sequencing information to inform NHS care and practices.

National Institute of Healthcare Research: https://www.nihr.ac.uk/

Improving the health of the nation through health and social care research. Discover new and current clinical trials and how this research is informing and improving practice.

Social Prescribing around the World: https://socialprescribingacademy.org.uk/media/1yeoktid/social-prescribing-around-the-world.pdf

This document outlines social prescribing developments and innovations across the world to improve health and wellbeing.

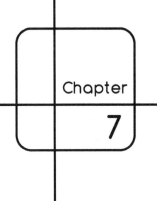

Case studies: Applying principles to practice

(Continued)

Part 1: Procedures to enable effective monitoring of a person's condition

1.1   accurately measure weight and height, calculate body mass index and recognise healthy ranges and clinically significant low/high readings.

Part 2: Procedures for provision of person-centred nursing care

4.3   record fluid intake and output to identify signs of dehydration or fluid retention and escalate as necessary.

10.2   undertake accurate drug calculations for a range of medications.

10.4   exercise professional accountability in ensuring safe administration of medicines to those receiving care.

Chapter aims

After reading this chapter, you will be able to:

- Apply theoretical knowledge of mathematical principles to situations in practice. Consider numeracy skills and drug calculations in context, understanding how it ties in with broader medicines management principles and safety measures.

Introduction

Patient safety reports indicate that around 10 per cent of all national reported incidents are due to medication errors, many of which could have been prevented (NHS Improvement, 2019). Moreover, medication errors are most likely at the administration phase, with drug calculation a key element of this process (WHO, 2017b). To be able to prevent these avoidable harms to patients, we must have an open reporting culture for medication errors and near misses to learn from them and improve patient safety (NHS Improvement, 2019). This is part of our professional duty as practitioners in accordance with the Nursing and Midwifery Council (NMC, 2018b). The NMC's role is to protect the public; therefore, sanctions can be imposed on staff if there are concerns regarding their fitness to practise. This highlights the need to maintain professional competence in medicines management, of which numeracy skills are a fundamental part. We have a duty to maintain knowledge and skills associated with all aspects of medicines administration, as well as to support each other in practice to check calculations and drug doses to ensure patient safety.

This final chapter is intended as a means for you to demonstrate the application of medicines management principles, allowing you to put the theory you have read within these chapters into practice and assure understanding of all the professional, legal and safe administration practices you have explored throughout this book.

The case studies that follow will allow you to reflect on safe administration and practise your numeracy skills. They are taken from across the fields of healthcare and the age continuum. As you are expected to work flexibly across the domains of nursing and in a wide range of settings as a qualified nursing associate, it is recommended that you work through all the case studies. This will develop your knowledge of medicines management principles from all areas of clinical practice, not just those you are familiar with.

To develop your confidence with these skills in practice, the following are the key drug calculation formulas you will need for clinical practice.

Formula reference sheet

It is a good idea to make a copy of these to have with you as a reference when calculating drugs in practice. Examples have been included with each formula. Please see Chapter 5 for further information about drug calculations and numeracy skills.

Converting units

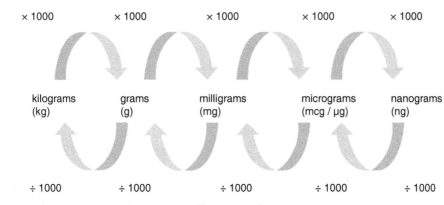

Figure 7.1   Converting large to small units and vice versa

Refer to Figure 7.1:

Convert 500mg paracetamol into grams (follow arrows):

500 ÷ 1000 = 0.5g paracetamol

Calculating number of tablets required

$$\frac{\text{What you want (prescribed amount)}}{\text{What you have got (dose available in stock)}} = \text{number of tablets required}$$

A patient is prescribed 30mg prednisolone, tablets in stock are 5mg:

30 ÷ 5 = 6 tablets required

Calculating solutions/injections

$$\frac{\text{What you want (prescribed amount)}}{\text{What you have got (dose available in stock)}} \times \text{volume (ml)}$$

Calpol (paracetamol oral suspension) is available as 120mg/5ml, the child is prescribed 60mg:

60 ÷ 120 × 5 = 2.5ml required

Calculating dose according to weight

Dose per kg × weight (kg) = personalised patient dose:

A child is prescribed co-amoxiclav 30mg/kg every 8 hours. They weigh 35kg.

30 x 35 = 1050mg (1.05g) needed every 8 hours

Calculating volume of fluid according to weight

0.5ml/kg/hr

0.5 × weight (kg) = ml per hour required

A patient weighs 70kg

0.5 × 70 = 35ml per hour required

Drip rate calculation

$$\frac{\text{volume (ml)} \times \text{drop factor (drops/ml)}}{\text{time (min)}} = \text{drops/min}$$

500ml IV fluid is prescribed over 5 hours; a regular giving set is used with a drop factor of 15 drops/ml

500 × 15 = 7500

5 × 60 = 300 minutes ∴ 7500 ÷ 300 = 25 drops/min

Flow rate calculation

Total volume ÷ time (hours) = ml per hour (flow rate)

A patient is prescribed 1000ml over 8 hours

1000 ÷ 8 = 125ml per hour

Case study 1: Muhammad

Muhammad recently suffered an ischaemic cerebral vascular accident (CVA) which has left him with severe left-sided weakness and limited mobility. He has dysphasia and dysphagia, communication and swallowing difficulties as a consequence of the stroke, as well as having a long-standing percutaneous endoscopic gastrostomy (PEG). His wife, Nadia, was taught how to administer his feed via the PEG before his discharge home.

On arriving at their home at 2 p.m., Nadia is glad to see you. The dietician has increased the speed of the feed and she would like you to run through the procedure with her again as she is anxious and fears that she has got the infusion rate wrong now that the prescription has changed. She is also concerned that the feed may be giving Muhammad diarrhoea. This has not been measured and his fluid balance chart (see Table 7.1) is also not up to date. Nadia can only tell you that he has had his bowels opened 5 times already today which is distressing for him and difficult to manage due to his poor mobility.

1 litre of feed ran overnight over 8 hours, finishing at 6am (as per the dietician's new regime). It is next due at 10pm.

Nadia tells you that Muhammad's morning medications were administered at 8 a.m. and 12.30 p.m. via the PEG along with flushes. His urinary catheter has not been emptied yet today; there is an accumulative total of 425ml. The following medications were administered:

Aspirin 300mg dispersible tablet OD. 150mg tablets are available in the cupboard.

Lactulose 15mg oral solution, the solution it comes in is 3mg/5ml BD.

Simvastatin 60mg oral suspension, which is available as 20mg/5ml OD.

1. Work out the infusion rate in accordance with the dietician's instructions.

2. Calculate the doses for Muhammad's medications:

   a) How many aspirin tablets were administered this morning?

   b) What was the volume of lactulose administered this morning?

   c) How much simvastatin solution was given?

3. A 50ml saline flush was given before the morning medication and afterwards, aspirin was dispersed into 10ml fluid and a 10ml flush was given between each medication. How much fluid in total was administered through the PEG to give Muhammad his morning medications?

4. Complete Muhammad's fluid balance with the information you have been given. Is it accurate?

5. What other information will you gather/consider? What actions will you take given the situation? Which professionals will you contact in relation to his care?

6. What factors will affect the absorption of his medications?

7. Why has Muhammad been prescribed syrups instead of tablets?

8. What does aspirin do to the body? What pharmacodynamic mechanism occurs?

Answers can be found at the end of this chapter.

Table 7.1   Fluid balance chart for case study 1: Muhammad

Date:

Hours	Input			Output			
	Oral intake	**IV fluids/ medication**	**Enteral feed**	**Urine**	**Stool**	**Vomit**	**Other**
01.00			125ml				
02.00			125ml				
03.00			125ml				
04.00			125ml				
05.00			125ml				
06.00			125ml				
07.00							
08.00			Pre-med 50ml flush 50ml medication + 20ml flush Post-meds 50ml flush				
09.00							
10.00							
11.00							
12.00							
13.00							
14.00				425ml catheter emptied	BO × 5		
15.00							
16.00							
17.00							
18.00							
19.00							
20.00							
21.00							
22.00							
23.00							
00.00							
Total							

Date:

Hours	Input			Output			
	Oral intake	**IV fluids/ medication**	**Enteral feed**	**Urine**	**Stool**	**Vomit**	**Other**
Total	?			?			
Fluid balance over 24hrs	?						

Case study 2: Adam

Adam is 41 years old and is currently in a Remand centre awaiting a decision regarding a criminal matter. Adam has disclosed to you that he takes opiates (heroin) illicitly and he acknowledges he has a high alcohol intake. He has been offered psychosocial interventions alongside his opioid substitution treatment of buprenorphine which he takes under direct supervision. He takes 4mg daily. He has been added to the 'unlock list' to attend the 'Meds hatch' for his other prescribed medications. He has his prison ID card and is instructed to take his medications in front of the dispenser. These include Thiamine supplements of 100mg daily as a divided dose of 50 mg bd, and as Adam also has insomnia from the altered living circumstances in the Remand centre he has been taking Zopiclone 7.5mg once a day at bedtime. The Thiamine hydrochloride is available as Athiam 100mg/5ml oral solution.

1. a) What volume of Athiam solution will you require to dispense morning and evening?

   b) What is the rationale for insisting Adam takes his medications in front of the dispenser?

   c) The Zopiclone is available as 3.75mg tablets, how many does Adam need at bedtime?

   d) The Buprenorphine strength you have available is 400 micrograms. How many tablets would Adam need? As his advocate what would you wish to discuss with the pharmacist dispensing?

   e) What is the schedule and class of Buprenorphine? What implications does this have for dispensing and administering?

Answers can be found at the end of this chapter.

Case study 3: Leon

You are a student nursing associate working with the Community Mental Health Team at their outpatient clinic. Leon has schizophrenia. He has been on the long-acting depot injection, fluphenazine decanoate, to manage his symptoms for many years. His usual dose is fluphenazine

(Continued)

(Continued)

62.5mg every 14 days. The anti-psychotic is available in stock as 25mg/ml or 100mg/ml. The nurse you have been working with has told you for safe administration that the depot injection (intramuscular ventrogluteal site) should not exceed 3ml in volume. Leon has recently started smoking again as his new girlfriend smokes. This has meant that his dose was adjusted at his last appointment, so his new dose is now 80mg every 14 days. Leon arrives for his appointment and tells you that he is experiencing more side effects than usual; he has been finding it difficult to sleep and has been feeling sick. He refuses to have the higher dose again today due to the side effects he is experiencing.

1. Calculate Leon's original dose.

2. a) Calculate his new adjusted dose using the stock solution 25mg/ml.

   b) Calculate his new adjusted dose using the stock solution 100mg/ml.

   c) Which stock solution will you use and why?

3. Calculate how many mg of fluphenazine Leon was having each month when he was taking his original dose.

4. Calculate how many mg more of fluphenazine Leon is having each month now his dose has been changed.

5. How does fluphenazine decanoate affect the body?

6. Why does smoking affect the dosing of this medication?

7. What action is needed given his situation?

8. Why is this medication given intramuscularly and through the ventrogluteal site?

Answers can be found at the end of this chapter.

Case study 4: Tracey

Tracey is a long-standing smoker who has asthma and depression. She has come for an asthma review at the surgery. You are shadowing the practice nurse. Tracey is on a combined long-acting beta2 agonist and inhaled corticosteroid, beclometasone with formoterol, x 2 inhalations twice daily. Tracey informs you that these are not very effective. She also takes theophylline 325mg every 12 hours. Tablets available are 175mg. She has recently been started on fluoxetine 20mg due to regular dips in her mood. These are available as 10mg tablets. During the discussion, Tracey states that she has lost her appetite over the last few weeks and has lost weight; she weighed herself this morning and she was 7 stone 8 pounds. You check in her notes and she is 1.68m in height and weighed 54kg three months ago.
  Spirometry is performed and her results are as follows:

Her forced expiratory volume (FEV) in 1 second is 2.23

Her forced vital capacity (FVC) is 3.98

A FEV:FVC ratio of less than 70 per cent indicates airflow obstruction (NICE, 2017b). The percentage can be calculated using the following equation:

$$\frac{FEV}{FVC} \times 100 = \%$$

1. Calculate Tracey's FEV:FVC ratio as a percentage (to the nearest whole number) using the equation above.

2. The practice nurse asks you to calculate Tracey's 'MUST' score (see Figure 7.2):

    a) Step 1: Calculate her BMI (to the nearest whole number) using today's weight.

    b) Step 2: Calculate the percentage of her unplanned weight loss in three months.

    c) Tracey scores 0 for Step 3 of the 'MUST' as she is not acutely unwell and is having some nutritional intake.

    d) Step 4: Calculate her final 'MUST' score.

    e) Step 5: What action is needed?

3. Look up the side effects of fluoxetine. Is Tracey experiencing any of these?

4. Look up the side effects of theophylline. What advice would you give Tracey in relation to this?

5. How many doses of theophylline does Tracey have each day?

6. Calculate how many fluoxetine tablets she needs per dose.

7. Tracey has identified that the inhalers she takes are not very effective. How do these different inhalers work and how might you advise her to optimise the effect of medication via this route?

Answers can be found at the end of this chapter.

Case study 5: Joel

Joel is 16 years old. He has autism spectrum disorder and attention deficit disorder. He takes atomoxetine 1200mcg/kg daily: 4mg/ml oral solution, given in two divided doses. He is 53kg. He has had a bad outbreak of eczema which has become infected and is weeping. The GP has prescribed him hydrocortisone 1 per cent with miconazole (10mg/gram hydrocortisone, 20mg/gram miconazole) which comes in a 30g tube. The GP has also written him up for Oilatum bath additive, 1–3 capfuls per bath, and Oilatum cream to use twice daily.

Joel's mum tells you that she is concerned about his mental health as he has been having suicidal thoughts.

1. Calculate the doses for Joel's medication:

    a) Calculate his daily dose of atomoxetine according to his weight.

    b) Calculate how much atomoxetine oral solution needs to be drawn up for each individual dose, to the nearest whole number.

    c) How many grams of steroid are there in a 30g tube?

    d) How many grams of antibacterial are there in a 30g tube?

(Continued)

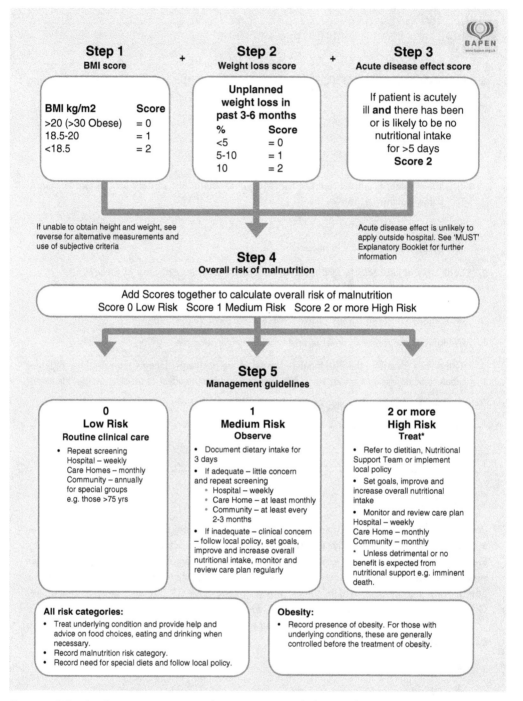

Figure 7.2 'Malnutrition Universal Screening Tool' ('MUST'). *Note:* Step 3 of the 'MUST' is unlikely to apply outside hospital (BAPEN, 2011).

Source: The 'Malnutrition Universal Screening Tool' ('MUST') is reproduced with the kind permission of BAPEN (British Association for Parenteral and Enteral Nutrition), 2011. For further information on 'MUST', see www.bapen.org.uk

2. To ensure concordance with his eczema treatment, how will you educate Joel and his mum about how to use these creams to maximise their effect? Look up guidance within the BNF.

3. What is the MHRA advice regarding emollients?

4. What are some of the possible side effects of atomoxetine?

5. How will you manage this situation in relation to the concerns raised by Joel's mum?

Answers can be found at the end of this chapter.

Case study 6: Catherine

Catherine is 12 years old and she weighs 53 pounds. She has cerebral palsy with associated muscle spasticity. She also has gastro-oesophageal reflux disease (GORD), swallowing and feeding difficulties. She has a naso-gastric (NG) feed, but can tolerate small amounts of thickened fluid. The NG feed is due (1500ml over 9 hours), but the tube has become blocked. When this is explored further, it turns out that Catherine's mum has not been flushing the line properly.

Catherine is on the following medications: omeprazole 40mg OD, 20mg tablets are available. Hyoscine hydrobromide transdermal patches to reduce hypersalivation, 1mg every 72 hours; each patch has 1mg of hyoscine hydrobromide. Baclofen, a muscle relaxer, 1.5mg/kg divided into 4 daily doses. It comes in a 5mg/5ml oral solution. Diazepam 10mg twice daily, oral solution 2mg/5ml. Ibuprofen, 400mg, 4 times a day, 100mg/5ml strawberry flavour. Domperidone 250mcg/kg 3 times a day for GERD, the oral solution comes as 1mg/ml. She also has daily increments of gabapentin. Today, she is due 15mg/kg 3 times a day, tomorrow she is due 20mg/kg 3 times a day. The solution comes in 50mg/ml solution.

1. Calculate Catherine's medications:
   a) How many omeprazole tablets does she need?

   b) How many days will 1 hyoscine hydrobromide patch last?

   c) Calculate what Catherine's baclofen daily dose is.

   d) How much baclofen is needed per dose?

   e) How much baclofen solution needs to be administered for 1 dose?

   f) Calculate how much diazepam solution needs to be administered for each dose.

   g) Calculate how much ibuprofen needs drawing up per dose.

   h) Calculate how much domperidone she needs per dose.

   i) How many ml of gabapentin need to be administered today for an individual dose?

   j) How many ml of gabapentin need to be administered tomorrow in total?

2. Calculate how many ml per hour the feed needs to run at (to the nearest whole number).

3. What are your actions in relation to the blocked feed? When should the NG be flushed?

Answers can be found at the end of this chapter.

Case study 7: Care quality commission survey

You are asked to compile some statistical data for the ward manager. It involves gathering information from the 2018 Adult Inpatient Survey (CQC, 2019).

178,681 people were sent questionnaires.

The response rate in 2018 was 45 per cent; in 2017, the response rate was 41 per cent.

80 per cent of respondents said they had always been treated with dignity and respect during their stay.

28 per cent stated they were not able to discuss their fears or concerns during their time in hospital; this has increased since last year (27 per cent in 2017). During the summer of 2018, bed occupancy was 90 per cent. Evidence suggests 85 per cent or more hospitals experience bed shortages and a higher prevalence of hospital-acquired infections because of this.

Two-thirds of people reported to be in pain while they were an inpatient in hospital, similar to rates in 2017; 67 per cent claimed that staff did everything they could to alleviate their pain.

41 per cent stated their discharge home was delayed and three-quarters of patients identified that this was due to waiting for medication.

15 per cent of people reported that they were not given clear written information about the medication they were discharged on. This has increased from last year when it was 13 per cent. Furthermore, 9 per cent felt that the medication they were discharged with was not clearly explained and it was unclear what its purpose was.

1. Calculate the increase in response rate from 2017 to 2018 as a percentage.

2. If 178,681 people were sent questionnaires and only 45 per cent responded, how many people took part in the study, to the nearest whole number?

3. If two-thirds of patients were in pain during their stay, what percentage would this be, to the nearest whole number?

4. If three-quarters of patients were delayed from going home due to waiting for medication, what percentage is this?

5. Consider the statistics in relation to pain management. How can these statistics be improved? What can you do within your role to address patient's pain more effectively?

6. Consider the statistics about information relating to medications. How can this be improved?

Answers can be found at the end of the chapter.

Case study 8: Bert

Bert is receiving palliative care as he has stage IV colon cancer which has metastasised to the liver. He has had bowel surgery, chemotherapy and stents due to a previous bowel obstruction. You are visiting him at home with the district nurse. He has noticeable ascites, which is making him breathless and jaundiced. He has been taking spironolactone tablets to reduce his ascites; these have recently been stopped as he is no longer able to swallow; fluid is beginning to build up in his abdomen.

Bert's current symptoms are nausea, intermittent confusion, pain and constipation. He is anaemic due to ongoing melaena. The syringe driver needs renewing. He is due diamorphine 40mg over 24 hours (5mg/ml solution for injection ampoule), levomepromazine 50mg/24 hours (ampoules for injection are 25mg/ml), midazolam 15mg/24 hours (ampoules come in 5mg/5ml), hyoscine hydrobromide 2mg/24 hours (400mcg/ml solution for injection ampoules) and diluted with water for injection.

Bert has an advanced care plan and DNR in place.

1. a) Calculate how much diamorphine needs drawing up for the syringe driver.

    b) Calculate how much levomepromazine needs drawing up.

    c) Calculate how much midazolam needs drawing up.

    d) Calculate how much hyoscine hydrobromide needs drawing up.

    e) If the syringe driver needs diluting up to 50ml with water for injection, how much dilution needs to be administered?

2. Why is the subcutaneous route used frequently in palliative care?

3. What checks will you do in relation to the syringe driver?

4. What are some of the possible side effects to taking diamorphine?

5. Are any of his medications hepatotoxic?

6. How does having metastatic liver disease and ascites impact on the pharmacodynamics of the drugs he is taking?

Outline answers can be found at the end of this chapter.

Case study 9: Sameer

Sameer is one of your patients on the Medical Assessment Unit due to symptoms of a urinary tract infection (UTI). He has suddenly deteriorated, spiking a temperature of 38.9°C and with steadily worsening cardiovascular observations. The medical team have reviewed him and the sepsis pathway has been commenced. He is 82kg.

Sameer is prescribed 500ml normal saline over 15 minutes (giving set drop factor 15), blood cultures are taken by the FY1, the following antibiotics are prescribed: IV piperacillin/tazobactam 4.5g 8hourly, IV gentamicin 3mg/kg reconstituted with 100ml 0.9 per cent sodium chloride over 30 minutes (once daily dose for 7 days). The dose should be rounded up/down to nearest 40mg. Gentamycin levels need to be checked 12 hours after the first dose to monitor concentration levels. If it is in the recommended range, 12 hours post initial dose serum gentamycin levels are < 2mg/L, then it is safe to give the next dose. Gentamycin levels can then be checked twice weekly along with full blood count. Ampoules are available in 80mg/2ml. Creatinine levels also require checking and a strict fluid balance observed.

The piperacillin comes in a powder with 2g piperacillin and 250mg tazobactam in each vial. It must be mixed well before adding to 100ml normal saline and be administered over 30 minutes. A colleague has found a Baxter pump to administer this through.

(Continued)

(Continued)

1. Calculate the drip rate for the IV fluids that have been prescribed.

2. How many vials of piperacillin/tazobactam are required?

3. Calculate the rate of infusion for the piperacillin/tazobactam.

4. Which three drugs need to be administered within an hour, in the Sepsis Six treatment regime?

5. Calculate how much gentamycin needs to be administered.

6. What side effects of gentamycin need to be monitored closely in this situation?

7. Why are gentamycin and creatinine levels checked following administration of gentamycin?

8. How does Sameer's obesity affect his treatment doses?

9. What type of antibiotics have been prescribed for Sameer?

10. Three days on, Sameer is experiencing bouts of diarrhoea. What are your priorities regarding this? Why has this happened?

Answers can be found at the end of this chapter.

Case study 10: Margaret

Margaret is 72 years old and has vascular dementia, she has long standing hypertension, hyperlipidaemia and type 2 diabetes mellitus, her current BMI is 25.8. She has had multiple TIA's and has had declining mobility and cognitive function in the last 5/6 years. This has affected her memory, mood and executive functions. She has recently been in hospital due to a chest infection, she has improved enough to be discharged, but there is a delay as she now needs an increased package of care. An MDT meeting has taken place including Margaret and her daughter who is her next of kin and main carer. It has been agreed she now needs to move to the specialist dementia care unit at the care home she is at, but there are no spaces currently. She has been moved to the intermediate care unit whilst she waits. Her most recent mini mental state exam scored 15/30, the last score recorded in her notes was 18/30, her BP 158/92mmHg. She is currently taking a wide range of medications including memantine, a NMDA receptor antagonist, antipsychotic medication, metformin. A target HbA1c level of 53mmol/mol (7.0%) has been agreed for managing her diabetes. You check her notes and her most recent level was at 58mmol/mol.

1. Calculate the percentage increase on Margaret's mini mental state exam score?

2. Use Diabetes UK conversion tool to identify what per cent Margarets most recent HbA1c level is at: **https://www.diabetes.org.uk/guide-to-diabetes/managing-your-diabetes/hba1c#converter**

3. What are the pharmacodynamics of the drug memantine?

4. Why is it important to involve Margaret in decisions about her care?

5. Can you think of any non-pharmacological interventions/support for Margaret, particularly in light of her co-morbidities and polypharmacy?

6. What percentage of decline has she had on her mini mental state exam (MMSE) score?

Answers can be found at the end of this chapter.

Case study 11: Sophie

Sophie is a six-year-old girl who has been rushed into A&E following an anaphylactic response after eating a sandwich that must have contained traces of nuts. She has been given adrenaline via her EpiPen, but is still exhibiting symptoms of respiratory distress, facial swelling, hypotension, tachycardia and a reduced level of consciousness. Her airway has been secured and 15l oxygen is being administered.

Adrenaline IM is in the ratio of 1:1000 (1mg/ml). Sophie is prescribed 150mcg adrenaline

You are asked by one of the team to draw up 5mg chlorphenamine to be given IV. The solution comes in vials of 10mg/ml. You draw up 2ml of chlorphenamine and the nurse administers it intravenously. Sophie is written up for 20ml/kg IV bolus.

1. a) What is happening physiologically in anaphylaxis?

    b) How does treatment improve the symptoms?

2. Calculate how much adrenaline needs to be administered.

3. a) How will you calculate Sophie's IV bolus without knowing her weight?

    b) Sophie's mum tells you that her daughter is about 19kg. Should you use this measure to calculate the dose?

4. a) Can you spot the drug error that has been made?

    b) How should you respond to this now that you have realised the error? What action should be taken?

    c) Whose responsibility is it?

Answers can be found at the end of this chapter.

Case study 12: Lydia

You are a trainee nursing associate working alongside a health visitor. You visit Lydia and her eight-week-old son Myles. Lydia tells you that Myles has become very unsettled the last few days and is not breast feeding well and it has also become very painful for her. He has had fewer wet and dirty nappies and Lydia is worried that he is not putting on weight. Two weeks ago he weighed 3.8kg, head circumference: 36cm and length: 52cm. She gets quite tearful when discussing this and says she is feeling a bit overwhelmed. Her antidepressants were swapped during pregnancy and she is wondering if she can restart her previous medication now that she has given birth as this seemed to work better. She was previously on paroxetine and is now on sertraline.

The health visitor asks you to weigh Myles, get a height and head circumference (3.85kg, 53cm and 36.2cm). On further discussion, it becomes clear that Myles has white spots on his tongue indicating thrush. He is prescribed nystatin and Lydia is prescribed miconazole cream and advised that she can take paracetamol or ibuprofen for the pain. Lydia says that she has been taking some co-codamol which has been helping.

(Continued)

(Continued)

Nystatin 100,000 units x 4 daily prescribed, to be given after feeds. Oral suspension available as 100,000 units/ml.

Daktarin 2 per cent, miconazole nitrate 20mg per gram, to be applied twice daily, continuing 10 days after lesions heal.

1. Calculate how much nystatin is needed per dose.

2. Why does Lydia also need to be treated for thrush?

3. If 2 per cent of the cream contains miconazole, how many mg is there in a 20mg tube?

4. Look up paroxetine and sertraline in the BNF. What is the advice around using this medication in pregnancy? Why was her antidepressant medication swapped at the start of her pregnancy?

5. Look up sertraline in LactMed: **https://toxnet.nlm.nih.gov/newtoxnet/lactmed.htm**. What is the advice about using sertraline when breastfeeding?

6. Are there benefits to Lydia continuing to breastfeed? If so, what are they?

7. Using the Royal College of Paediatrics and Child Health (RCPCH) growth chart, **www.rcpch.ac.uk/sites/default/files/Boys_0-4_years_growth_chart.pdf**, calculate which centile Myles was for his weight, height and head circumference two weeks ago.

8. Calculate which centile Myles is on today for his weight, height and head circumference. What does this indicate?

Answers can be found at the end of this chapter.

Case study 13: Maternity survey

You are asked to investigate some statistical data to enhance your understanding of an aspect of health care. It involves gathering information from the maternity survey (CQC, 2022c). The survey looked at experiences of pregnant people who had a live birth in early 2022 with 20,927 people who had recently given birth being sent questionnaires.

Since 2017 there has been a positive upward trend from 55 per cent to 62 per cent of no delay in the discharge from hospital.

Three quarters said their midwife asked about their mental health during antenatal care.

85 per cent said they were given enough mental health support, and in 2021, this had been 83 per cent.

Two thirds reported 'definitely' having confidence and trust in staff delivering their antenatal care.

A fifth said there were not offered any choices about where to have their baby.

An inequality in maternal mortality and neonatal deaths were recorded. The lowest still birth rates were for babies of white ethnicity from the least deprived areas, compared with the highest rates for babies of black African and black Caribbean ethnicity from the most deprived areas (8 per 1000 total births). Readmission in the post-partum period differed as well. 102 per 1000 for black women compared with 74 re-admissions per 1000 for white women.

Staffing levels had altered with 26,556 midwives in July 2021 and 26,041 in July 2022. This coincides with a National birth rate of 624,828 live births in England and Wales in 2021. The birth rate in 2022 was 613,936.

1. There has been a positive upward trend since 2017 in people receiving no delay in their discharge from hospital. What is this increase expressed as a percentage?

2. $^{3}/_{4}$ of respondents had been asked about their Mental health in the antenatal period, if 20,000 people responded to the questionnaire, how many had been asked about their Mental Health?

3. A fifth of respondents did not have a choice of where to deliver, how many people is this based on a respondent number of 20,000?

4. What is 102 per 1000 births as a percentage? What is 74 per 1000 births as a percentage? What is the difference between these figures as an indication of inequality pertaining to maternal re-admission?

5. What is the difference in the number of Midwives between July 2021 and July 2022?

6. What is the difference in the number of births in England and Wales between 2021 and 2022?

7. On reflection what are the implications of a reduction in Midwife numbers and the inequalities in health care provision for different service users' groups?

Answers can be found at the end of the chapter.

Chapter summary

This chapter has provided a range of practical-based scenarios that require drug calculations to practise numeracy skills. Having read through the different topics of this book, this chapter allows you to apply the knowledge you have gained of medicines management. To ensure safe administration of medication, healthcare professionals not only require expertise in numeracy and drug calculations but also an understanding of wider contextual or environmental factors such as pharmacology, pathophysiology, professional responsibilities and clinical skills. These scenarios draw on all of these elements to practise drug calculations within the context of practice situations that can often be complex and challenging. Practising these scenarios will not only increase confidence administering medication safely and avoiding any errors but also help to draw on wider knowledge to make appropriate clinical decisions to keep patients safe.

Case studies: Brief outline answers

Case study 1: Muhammad (page 6)

1. Work out the infusion rate in accordance with the dietician's instructions.
   1000ml ÷ 8 = **125ml per hour**

2. Calculate the doses for Muhammad's medications:

   a) aspirin: 300 ÷ 150 = **2 tablets**

   b) lactulose: 15 ÷ 3 × 5 = **25ml**

   c) simvastatin: 60 ÷ 20 × 5 = **15ml**

3. If a 50ml saline flush was given before the morning medication and afterwards, aspirin was dispersed into a 10ml fluid and a 10ml flush was given between each medication. How much fluid in total was administered through the PEG to give Muhammad his morning meds?
   50ml + 10ml + 10ml + 25ml + 10ml + 15ml + 50ml = **170ml**

4. Complete Muhammad's fluid balance with the information you have been given. Is it accurate?

   The fluid balance chart is not accurate as fluid lost in bowel movements has not been recorded.

5. What other information will you gather/consider? What actions will you take given the situation? Which professionals will you contact in relation to his care?

   Muhammad's case study demonstrates why it is important that fluid balance charts are completed accurately to monitor and assess the patient effectively. Muhammad does not seem to be tolerating the feed, which may be due to the speed of administration, in which case the dietician needs to review the regime. The case worker (district nurse) also needs to be informed. IV fluids may be needed to replenish losses and rebalance electrolytes due to the episodes of diarrhoea. A full assessment is required, particularly vital signs, which will give an indication of circulatory volume status. A stool sample should also be taken to identify if there is any infection. Lactulose is a laxative that draws water into the bowel to soften stools, so it is not indicated as Muhammad has diarrhoea. If medication is omitted for any reason, it should be clearly documented within the plan of care and the case worker informed.

6. What factors will affect the absorption of his medications?

   Gastrointestinal absorption through the PEG enters the stomach immediately. Liquid medicinal products are also generally quicker to absorb than solid formulations. However, the medications' bioavailability may be lowered because Muhammad has diarrhoea, as the medication may pass too quickly through the GI tract to be fully absorbed.

7. Why has Muhammad been prescribed syrups instead of tablets?

   Muhammad has difficulty swallowing tablets due to his dysphagia. Medication should not be altered without guidance from a pharmacist. If the drug is altered through crushing/splitting tablets or opening capsules, it can change the way the medication is absorbed, can alter the dose or cause irritation due to removing the protective coating on a tablet.

8. What does aspirin do to the body? What pharmacodynamic mechanism occurs?

   Aspirin binds to plasma proteins (albumin). If Muhammad becomes mal-nourished, he is at higher risk of a bleed as he will have less circulating plasma protein, leaving free unbound medicine in the bloodstream able to exert a medicinal effect.

Table 7.2 Completed fluid balance chart for Case study 1: Muhammad

Date:

Hours	Output			Output			
	Oral intake	**IV fluids/ medication**	**Enteral feed**	**Urine**	**Stool**	**Vomit**	**Other**
01.00			125ml				
02.00			125ml				
03.00			125ml				
04.00			125ml				
05.00			125ml				
06.00			125ml				
07.00							
08.00			Pre-med 50ml flush + 50ml medication + 20ml flush + 50ml post-meds flush				
09.00							
10.00							
11.00							
12.00							
13.00							
14.00				425ml catheter emptied	BO × 5		
15.00							
16.00							
17.00							
18.00							
19.00							
20.00							
21.00							
22.00							
23.00							
00.00							
Total							
Total	920ml			425ml			
Fluid balance over 24hrs	+ive fluid balance 495ml						
	Inaccurate as bowel movements have not been recorded.						

Case study 2: Adam (page 10)

1. a) What volume of Athiam solution will you require to dispense morning and evening?
    2.5ml

    b) What is the rationale for insisting Adam takes his medications in front of the dispenser?

    There is a chance that he may not comply with the regime and potentially keep medications back for self-harm or as a resource.

    c) The Zopiclone is available as 3.75mg tablets, how many does Adam need at bedtime?

    2 tablets

    d) The Buprenorphine strength you have available is 400 micrograms. How many tablets would Adam need? As his advocate what would you wish to discuss with the pharmacist dispensing?

    10 tablets, even though 400 microgram tablets are cheaper and aid small adjustments to be made on sliding scales 10 tablets is too many for Adam to take in one go and risks him keeping some back potentially.

    e) What is the schedule and class of Buprenorphine? What implications does this have for dispensing and administering?

    Schedule 3, Class C Controlled drug, organisational policy and procedures to maintain when procuring, prescribing and administering them, in line with Misuse of Drugs Act 1971.

Case study 3: Leon (page 11)

1. Calculate Leon's original dose.
    $62.5 \div 25 \times 1 = 2.5ml$

2. a) Calculate his new adjusted dose using the stock solution 25mg/ml.
    $80mg \div 25 \times 1 = 3.2ml$

    b) Calculate his new adjusted dose using the stock solution 100mg/ml.
    $80 \div 100 \times 1 = 0.8ml$

    c) Which stock solution will you use and why?

    100mg/ml as the weaker solution would involve giving a 3.2ml injection, which exceeds the recommended volume for the route of administration.

3. Calculate how many mg of fluphenazine Leon was having each month when he was taking his original dose.

    $62.5 \times 2 = 125mg$ per month with his original dose

4. Calculate how many mg more of fluphenazine Leon is having each month now his dose has been changed.

    125mg previously, $80 \times 2 = 160mg$ currently
    $\therefore 160 - 125 = 35mg$ more each month

5. How does fluphenazine decanoate affect the body?

Fluphenazine is an antipsychotic medication that is an antagonist that blocks dopamine receptors. Dopamine is transported through the mesolimbic system; this pathway regulates our reward, motivation and cognitive responses. By blocking dopamine receptors, it reduces dopamine excitability. This helps to reduce positive symptoms such as excess thought processes, such as hallucinations or delusions, as well as negative symptoms – that is, deficits such as depression. It is often more successful in treating positive rather than negative symptoms. Although it is less sedative and less antimuscarinic, it is more likely to cause extra pyramidal systems such as dyskinesia, dystonia and parkinsonism (Mersey Care, 2017).

6. Why does smoking affect the dosing of this medication?

Tobacco contains carcinogens that activate liver enzymes causing them to metabolise the medication more quickly, the induction of these enzymes means that there are lower plasma concentrations of the drug. Therefore, if a patient starts smoking, the medication will have reduced potency and vice versa. This is the reason why Leon's dose was adjusted.

7. What action is needed given his situation?

The procedure cannot take place without consent from the patient. More information is needed about the side effects he is experiencing and their severity, as this will impact on his treatment plan. This medication is known to cause extra pyramidal symptoms – that is, motor and coordination control, which can be very distressing and disabling for patients (BNF Online (https://bnf.nice.org.uk/): Psychoses and related disorders). Rating scales can be useful in assessing the severity and cause of side effects with antipsychotic medication. This information can then be passed on to the prescriber so they can decide whether a lower dose can be prescribed and administered safely. Smoking increases the clearance of fluphenazine, which is why Leon's dose was increased to obtain the therapeutic effect needed to control his symptoms. His dose needs to be titrated to minimise side effects from the medication, but also achieve the therapeutic effect required to treat his schizophrenia.

8. Why is this medication given intramuscularly and through the ventrogluteal site?

This is an oil-based deep intramuscular injection. The ventrogluteal site is identified within the research as one of the safest sites for IM injections as it is situated in deep muscle (glutaeus medius and glutaeus minimus) away from major blood vessels and nerves (Clinical Skills.net). It is a slow-release, long-acting medication. It takes 48–96 hours for the medication to affect psychotic symptoms and can last for over a month. This medication has a slow release with a half-life of plasma clearance of between two weeks to four months. This explains why Leon is prescribed the medication fortnightly. Having the IM injections twice weekly also improves compliance for those who may refuse or forget to take oral medication. To ensure appropriate absorption of the medication and to avoid subcutaneous injection, the size of needle must also be considered.

Case study 4: Tracey (page 13)

1. Calculate Tracey's FEV:FVC ratio as a percentage to the nearest whole number using the equation above.

$2.23 \div 3.98 \times 100 = 56\%$ indicating airflow obstruction

2. The practice nurse asks you to calculate Tracey's 'MUST' score (see Figure 7.2):

   a) Step 1: calculate her BMI (to the nearest whole number) using today's weight.

      1 stone = 6.35kg 6.35 × 7.8 = 49.53kg 50kg to the nearest whole number
      50kg ÷ (1.68 × 1.68) = 17.715 BMI 18
      ∴ step 1 = 2

   b) Step 2: calculate the percentage of unplanned weight loss in three months.

      Previously 54kg, now 50kg: 54 − 50 = 4kg loss in 3 months
      ∴ 4/54 × 100 = 7.4074...
      ∴ 7% unplanned weight loss
      ∴ step 2 = 1

   c) Step 3: Tracey scores 0 of the 'MUST' as she is not acutely unwell and is having some nutritional intake.

   d) Step 4: Calculate her final 'MUST' score.

      Tracey's final 'MUST' score: 2 + 1 = 3

   e) Step 5: what action is needed?

      As per 'MUST' screening tool, nutritional needs must be monitored and reviewed regularly, a care plan for nutrition instigated, as well as further assessments and investigations such as blood tests and vital signs.

3. Look up the side effects of fluoxetine. Is Tracey experiencing any of these?

   Affective disorders are characterised by disturbance of mood and associated with alterations in behaviour, energy, appetite, sleep and weight. Changes to appetite, altered taste and weight changes are all common side effects of fluoxetine. Adverse effects such as diarrhoea and nausea can also have a knock-on effect on nutritional status. This is likely to be the reason why Tracey has recently been losing weight. Fluoxetine is a selective serotonin reuptake inhibitor (SSRI) that binds to plasma proteins. If she is malnourished and has less plasma proteins, there will be greater amounts of unbound drug exerting a greater therapeutic effect. This may increase the potency of the drug and increase side effects. Furthermore, it has a long half-life and can take 5–6 weeks to be fully eliminated from the body. If side effects are present, they may also linger on after treatment stops.

4. Look up the side effects for theophylline. What advice would you give Tracey in relation to this?

   Tracey may not be aware that smoking reduces the efficacy of theophylline. It will also exacerbate her asthma symptoms. Have smoking cessation options been discussed with her?

5. How many doses of theophylline does Tracey have each day?
   24 ÷ 12 = 2 doses per day

6. Calculate how many fluoxetine tablets she needs per dose.
   20mg ÷ 10mg = 2 tablets

7. Tracey has identified that the inhalers she takes are not very effective. How do these different inhalers work and how might you advise her to optimise the effect of medication via this route?

   Tracey is taking a combined long-acting beta2 agonist and inhaled corticosteroid.

Formoterol acts by dilating the bronchioles and activates the same receptors as adrenaline, which is why palpitations can be a common side effect. Beclomethasone is the inhaled corticosteroid, which reduces inflammation within the airways by inhibiting inflammatory mediators. They are preventor inhalers to prevent flare-ups. It is important to take this medication even if the patient is not having symptoms. It is crucial that patients are aware of this to increase medication concordance. If there are concerns regarding the inhalers' effectiveness, it is also important to check her inhaler technique.

The inhalation route enables a rapid response at the desired site of action, which are the lungs. However, research suggests that three-quarters of patients are not using their inhalers correctly (Global Initiative for Asthma, 2019). Spacers can help to ensure that the drug is administered more effectively as the drug contents are locked into the chamber rather than being lost into the atmosphere. Another way of improving inhaler technique is through educating the patient about how to optimise the inhalation route. This includes advice regarding breathing, such as a full exhalation beforehand and holding the breath on release of the inhaler (Normansell et al., 2017).

The patient should also be offered smoking cessation at every opportunity to improve her symptoms. Smoking can reduce the effect of corticosteroid treatment, which Tracey may not be aware of.

Case study 5: Joel (page 15)

1. Calculate the doses for Joel's medication:

   a) Calculate Joel's daily dose of atomoxetine according to his weight.
      1200mcg = 1.2mg
      1.2 × 53 = **63.6mg**

   b) Calculate how much atomoxetine oral solution needs to be drawn up for each individual dose, to the nearest whole number.
      63.6 ÷ 4mg × 1 = 15.9ml total daily dose 15.9 ÷ 2 = 7.95 **8ml for each individual dose**

   c) How many grams of steroid are there in a 30g tube?
      10mg hydrocortisone in 1g 10 × 30 = **300mg in 30g of cream**
      (the 1 per cent refers to the potency of this steroid)

   d) How many grams of antibacterial are there in a 30g tube?
      20mg miconazole in 1g 20 × 30 = **600mg in 30g of cream**

2. To ensure concordance with his eczema treatment, how will you educate Joel and his mum about how to use these creams to maximise their effect? Look up guidance within the BNF.

As Joel has a learning need, it is important that his mum is also involved in treatment information to ensure medicines concordance. It is important that the emollient cream is used twice daily, even if his eczema has improved, to help prevent future outbreaks. This should be applied after washing to maximise absorption. Cream should be applied using a clean utensil such as a spoon. As Joel has a fungal infection, it is important that his regular emollient cream does not become contaminated. To maximise absorption, it should be applied in the same direction his hair is growing. The Oilatum bath additive he is prescribed can be applied to wet skin, so can also be used in the shower. These act as substitutes for soap to hydrate the skin. This additive should also be used as part of his daily routine, even when flare-ups have resolved.

Hydrocortisone and miconazole cream should be administered at a different time to the emollient to ensure full absorption. The steroid and antifungal should be applied thinly. Although this is a mild dose of steroid, if it is applied too thickly there can be a rebound effect when treatment stops. As it is a mild dose, it can be applied to the face for a short period of time (maximum seven days); stronger doses are not recommended for the face as it can thin the skin if overused.

3.   What is the MHRA advice regarding emollients?

The MHRA have released a warning regarding emollient use (both paraffin and non-paraffin emollients) due to the risk of burns. Emollients can seep through clothing and then catch alight if exposed to a naked flame such as smoking or cooking as it is highly flammable. Patients should be advised about this risk.

4.   What are some of the possible side effects of atomoxetine?

Atomoxetine can increase symptoms of depression and suicidal thoughts. This is particularly pertinent given the concerns that Joel's mum has raised at this appointment.

5.   How will you manage this situation in relation to the concerns raised by Joel's mum?

Her concerns regarding his mental health require further investigation to maintain patient safety and ensure that he receives the support he needs. A more in-depth psychological assessment is needed, screening tools such as the Patient Health Questionnaire and measure for Generalised Anxiety Disorder (PHQ9 and GAD7) are useful for gathering further information and understanding the level of risk to the patient and others, and help form an appropriate action plan for the patient. As identified within the previous question, one of the side effects of his ADHD medication is depression and suicidal thoughts, so this should be discussed with Joel and his mum. It is unclear how long he has been having these feelings and the cause of them, so this needs to be clarified. A medication review to consider alternative medication may be indicated. Referral to the mental health team is required as Joel may benefit from talking therapies, medication to help manage his mood or a combination of both.

Case study 6: Catherine (page 16)

1.   Calculate Catherine's medications:

a)   How many omeprazole tablets does she need?
$40 \div 20 = $ **2 tablets**

b)   How many days will 1 hyoscine hydrobromide patch last?
72 hours $\div$ 24 hours = **3 days**

c)   Calculate what Catherine's baclofen daily dose is.
1 pound = 0.45kg $\quad 0.45 \times 53 = $ 23.85kg
$\therefore$ 24kg (to the nearest whole number)
$1.5 \times 24 = $ **36mg total daily dose**

d) How much baclofen is needed per dose?

36 ÷ 4 = **9mg**

e) How much baclofen solution needs to be administered for 1 dose?

9 ÷ 5 × 5 = **9ml**

f) Calculate how much diazepam solution needs to be administered for each dose.

10 ÷ 2 × 5 = **25ml**

g) Calculate how much ibuprofen needs drawing up per dose.

400mg ÷ 100 × 5 = **20ml**

h) Calculate how much domperidone she needs per dose.

250mcg × 24kg = 6000mcg or 6mg

∴ 6mg ÷ 1 × 1 = **6mg 3 times a day**

i) How many ml of gabapentin need to be administered today for an individual dose?

15 × 24 = 360mg

∴ 360 ÷ 50 × 1 = **7.2ml per dose**

j) How many ml of gabapentin need to be administered tomorrow in total?

20 × 24 = 480ml

∴ 480 ÷ 50 × 1 = 9.6ml per dose

∴ 9.6 × 3 = **28.8ml over 3 divided doses**

2. Calculate how many ml per hour the feed needs to run at, to the nearest whole number?

1500 ÷ 9 = 166.666666 ... **167ml per hour**

3. What are your actions in relation to the blocked feed? When should the NG be flushed?

The tube will need to be unblocked by administering 30–50ml water to flush or withdraw contents. It is important to discuss with Catherine's mum when flushes need to be administered. As she has a range of medication in syrup form, the NG tube will block again if it is not being flushed regularly. Guidelines suggest 50ml before and after feeds and 10ml between each medication that is administered

Case study 7: Care Quality Commission Survey (page 18)

1. Calculate the increase in response rate from 2017 to 2018 as a percentage?

45 − 41 = **4%**

2. If 178,681 people were sent questionnaires and only 45 per cent responded, how many people took part in the study, to the nearest whole number?

45 ÷ 100 × 178,681 = **80,406 participated**

3. If two-thirds of patients were in pain during their stay, what percentage would this be, to the nearest whole number?

2 ÷ 3 = 0.6666...

∴ 0.66 × 100 = 66.6666...

∴ **67%**

4. If three-quarters of patients were delayed from going home due to waiting for medication, what percentage is this?

   $3 \div 4 = 0.75$

   $\therefore 0.75 \times 100 = 75\%$

5. Consider the statistics in relation to pain management. How can these statistics be improved? What can you do within your role to address patients' pain more effectively?

   Two-thirds of patients experienced pain whilst being an in-patient. Furthermore, 33 per cent felt nursing staff could have done more to alleviate their pain. This can be addressed by acknowledging the subjectivity of pain and ensuring that we are checking pain scores regularly. It is also important to draw on the observations of our patients to identify pain, raised respiratory rate or heart rate, which can indicate pain, as well as their behaviour. Although pain assessment is not part of the NEWS2 observation chart, it is acknowledged by the Royal College of Physicians (2017) that it should be measured alongside physiological parameters to provide a broader clinical picture of how well the patient is doing. Another way in which this can be addressed is by ensuring that patients are prescribed appropriate analgesia. The WHO (1986) pain ladder recommends a stepped approach to managing pain drawing on different types of analgesia depending on its severity. The more we know about the type of pain a patient is experiencing, the easier it is to ensure appropriate analgesia. For instance, breakthrough analgesia may be required for severe intermittent pain and slow-release medication may be indicated more for chronic pain. The right drug, route, dose and time are crucial to ensure that pain is managed effectively. For more information on pain management, see Chapter 6.

6. Consider the statistics about information relating to medications. How can this be improved?

   A total of 75 per cent of patients who had a delayed discharge identified that this was because of waiting for medication. Although discharge planning and To Take Out (TTO) medication is a joined-up multidisciplinary process, TNAs can help to enhance efficiency in this area through planning discharge when a patient is first admitted. Clear communication with other professionals during ward rounds and MDT meetings help to ensure that patients are on the appropriate medication to return home with. TNAs also have a crucial role in ensuring that patients fully understand the medication they have been started on in order to take it as intended. This report highlights the need for both verbal and written information for patients regarding their medication to make sure that information is clear and remembered on discharge.

Case study 8: Bert (page 19)

1. Calculate how much medication needs drawing up for the syringe driver.

   a) Diamorphine:

   $40 \div 5 \times 1 = 8ml$ over 24 hours

   b) Levomepromazine:

   $50 \div 25 \times 1 = 2ml$ over 24 hours

c) Midazolam:

15 ÷ 5 × 5 = 15ml over 24 hours

d) Hyoscine hydrobromide:

2mg = 2000mcg

∴ 2000 ÷ 400 × 1 = 5ml over 24 hours

e) If the syringe driver needs diluting up to 50ml with water for injection, how much dilution needs to be administered?

8 + 2 + 15 + 5 = 30ml

∴ 50 − 30ml = 20ml water for injection needed

2. Why is the subcutaneous route used frequently in palliative care?

Commonly, it is because they are unable to swallow or take medication orally and it allows continuous delivery of medication to manage a range of symptoms. Syringe drivers allow multiple medications to be administered at the same time for a longer duration and avoid frequent injections, which are uncomfortable for patients.

3. What checks will you do in relation to the syringe driver?

The infusion site must be checked regularly and may need to be moved if it becomes swollen, inflamed or sore. Regular monitoring of the infusion is needed to check that medication is infusing correctly as per the rate of infusion and there are no occlusions. Side effects of the medication must be monitored, as well as the patient's symptoms to ensure that it is effective

4. What are some of the possible side effects to taking diamorphine?

Although it may improve Bert's pain, it may increase some of his other symptoms such as nausea, vomiting and confusion. He is taking midazolam and diamorphine, which both have sedatory effects, so this should be monitored closely. Furthermore, opioids may increase the risk of encephalopathy. This may be the cause of his confusion as he has metastatic liver disease. Encephalopathy can be a complication of liver disease as the failing organ is not able to detoxify waste products such as ammonia, as it would normally do, so toxins can build up in the bloodstream and cause damage. Opioids can improve breathlessness, which may be beneficial for Bert.

5. Are any of his medications hepatotoxic?

Diamorphine should be used with caution in hepatic impairment for reasons detailed above. Midazolam is not recommended for patients with hepatic impairment. However, it does have a shorter half-life; therefore, it is processed more quickly than other benzodiazepines, so it is safer than other alternatives.

6. How does having metastatic liver disease and ascites impact on the pharmacodynamics of the drugs he is taking?

Bert's ascites has caused albumin to leak into his abdomen (due to portal hypertension), which has caused serum albumin to reduce. Therefore, the medication has less plasma proteins to bind to, increasing the therapeutic effect and the potency of the drugs. The liver metastases have caused hepatic failure. This therefore means that drug metabolism is impaired, increasing the toxicity of the medication administered. Furthermore, hepatic failure can also gradually impact on renal functioning as well, so elimination of the medication may also be affected.

Case study 9: Sameer (page 21)

1. Calculate the drip rate for the IV fluids that have been prescribed.
   50ml × 15 drop factor ÷ 15 (mins) = **50 drops per min**

2. How many vials of piperacillin/tazobactam are required?
   4.5g prescribed
   2000mg piperacillin + 250mg tazobactam = 2250mg or 2.25g × 2 = 4.5g
   2 vials needed

3. Calculate the rate of infusion for the piperacillin/tazobactam.
   100ml over 30 mins = 3.333ml per min (3ml per minute) or 200ml per hour

4. Which three drugs need to be administered within an hour in the Sepsis Six treatment regime?
   IV fluid, broad-spectrum IV antibiotics and high flow oxygen if needed

5. Calculate how much gentamycin needs to be administered.
   3 mg × 82 kg = 246 to the nearest 40mg. 246 ÷ 40 = 6.15
   ∴ 40 × 6 = 240mg (dose rounded down to nearest 40mg)
   240 ÷ 80 × 2 = 6ml **gentamycin reconstituted into 100ml normal saline**

6. What side effects of gentamycin need to be monitored closely in this situation?

   Side effects are related to dosing, hence the reason that gentamycin is closely measured and monitored. Gentamycin can increase the risk of acute kidney injury (AKI). Gentamycin is mostly processed within the kidneys. It is contraindicated in renal impairment, as if the drug is not excreted adequately by the kidneys, it will cause toxicity. Low urine output is one of the classifications for AKI, along with raised creatinine levels. This needs to be monitored closely and more IV fluids need prescribing to resuscitate the patient.

7. Why are gentamycin and creatinine levels checked following administration of gentamycin?

   This drug has a very narrow therapeutic window. It needs an initial high dose to create a peak concentration that will kill the bacteria and then levels should drop to minimise the risk of side effects. Gentamycin has an after effect of preventing growth of bacteria, so lower doses can be used that still have a good therapeutic effect.
   Large doses can be toxic to the kidneys and can cause deafness if overdosed, so it is important to monitor renal function and dose levels closely to avoid serious side effects.

8. How does Sameer's obesity affect his treatment doses?

   The distribution of gentamycin is affected because of his obesity. Gentamycin distributes poorly through fat tissue, meaning that obese patients need a lower dose.

9. What type of antibiotics have been prescribed for Sameer?

   Piperacillin tazobactam is a beta-lactam, a broad-spectrum antibiotic that kills bacteria through inhibiting growth of the bacteria cell wall (bacteriocidal). Piperacillin/tazobactam works by breaking down the cell wall so that gentamycin can get inside the bacterial cell and inhibit protein synthesis that is needed for the bacteria to replicate and survive.

10. Three days on, Sameer is experiencing bouts of diarrhoea. What are your priorities regarding this? Why has this happened?

Broad-spectrum antibiotics such as the ones Sameer has been taking can damage the gut microbiome leading to antibiotic-associated colitis and increased risk of Clostridium difficile. Therefore, a sample must be taken to identify any infection. Strict infection control must be maintained to avoid the spread of infection. Sameer's initial blood cultures will have come back by now and he should be put on specific antibiotics to kill the specific microorganism that caused his infection. This is important in order to treat the infection as quickly and appropriately as possible, as well as to maintain antibiotic stewardship.

Case study 10: Margaret (page 22)

1. Calculate the percentage increase on Margaret's mini mental state exam score?
$18 - 15 = 3$
$3/30 \times 100 = 10\%$

2. Use Diabetes UK conversion tool to identify what per cent Margarets most recent HbA1c level is at:
$58\text{mmol/mol} = 7.5\%$

3. What are the pharmacodynamics of the drug memantine?

Evidence suggests that overactivity/damage to excitatory neurotransmitters (glutamate) in the central nervous system, particularly at NMDA receptors, occurs in patients with advancing dementia and leads to some of the more debilitating symptoms associated with this condition. Memantine, an NMDA receptor antagonist, inhibits the action of glutamate at these receptors specifically, which has been found to improve cognitive and physical functioning, with improvements in MMSE scores over as little as six months. Although improvements in symptoms have been identified, it has not been found to prevent or delay neurodegeneration. See medicines.org.uk/drugbank UK for further information.

4. Why is it important to involve Margaret in decisions about her care?

As part of ensuring a person-centred delivery of care, Margaret needs to be involved in decisions about her care, in line with the Mental Capacity Act (2005). She may well have been assessed as not having capacity, but this does not mean she should not still be involved in decision-making. Information may need to be tailored to her needs and delivered in different ways to aid understanding, for instance, visual aids.

5. Can you think of any non-pharmacological interventions/support for Margaret, particularly in light of her co-morbidities and polypharmacy?

Occupational therapy for cognitive rehabilitation, social support/activities within the home, social prescribing, dietary and lifestyle interventions to address her diabetes, hyperlipidaemia and hypertension.

6. What percentage of decline has she had on her mini mental state exam (MMSE) score?

$15/30 = 0.5$
$18/30 = 0.6$
10% decline in MMSE score

Case study 11: Sophie (page 22)

1. a) What is happening physiologically in anaphylaxis?

    Anaphylaxis is a systemic (whole body) response to an allergen and is a medical emergency. Systemic treatment is needed to treat life-threatening symptoms compromising the airway, breathing and or circulation, using the A–E assessment (Resuscitation Council, 2021a, 2021b). The hypersensitive immune response causes inflammatory markers to be released such as histamine, causing vasodilation and increased permeability of blood vessels and vasoconstriction of the bronchioles. This has led to Sophie's low blood pressure and difficulty breathing. Please see Resus Council in the Useful websites section below for full guidelines on the treatment of anaphylaxis.

    b) How does treatment improve symptoms?

    Adrenaline stimulates both alpha- and beta-adrenergic receptors, stimulation of alpha receptors cause vasoconstriction, increasing cardiac output and therefore blood pressure (EMC, n.d.). Stimulation of beta receptors allows the bronchioles to dilate, opening the airways and preventing further inflammatory mediators being released. It is administered IM or IV to enable fast action as life-threatening symptoms of anaphylaxis develop fast.

2. Calculate how much adrenaline needs to be administered.
    Adrenaline is given in the ratio 1:1000 (1mg/ml)
    150mcg adrenaline prescribed = 0.15mg
    0.15mg: 0.15ml
    0.15ml

3. a) How will you calculate Sophie's IV bolus without knowing her weight?

    There are numerous ways to estimate a child's weight in emergency situations. There is the Broseley paediatric emergency tape for height measurement and therefore weight estimation in emergency situations. There is the PAWPER (Paediatric Advanced Weight Prediction in the Emergency Room) which measures length and girth/frame. There is also the Mercy Tape (taking the guesswork out of paediatric weight estimation) using length and circumference of the upper arm. See Further reading for more information on these measures.

    b) Sophie's mum tells you that she is roughly 19kg. Should you use this measure to calculate the dose?

    It is more accurate to use one of the measuring assessment tools discussed above. These are evidence-based tools.

4. a) Can you spot the drug error that has been made?

    Sophie is prescribed 5mg chlorphenamine; vials of 10mg/ml are available.
    5 ÷ 10 × 1 = 0.5ml not 2ml

    b) How should you respond to this now that you have realised the error? What action should be taken?

    First, it is crucial we are honest about mistakes and alert senior staff as soon as possible to minimise harm to the patient. Reporting a drug error must follow your Trust policy and report system. This means that the situation can be investigated and learning can be gained from it. The Royal Pharmaceutical Society (RPS) (2020) recommends the following approach: Report, Learn, Share, Act and Review.

c) Whose responsibility is it?

RPS (2023) guidelines state that registered healthcare staff are responsible for their actions, mistakes and omissions in relation to medication administration and must always act with professionalism.

The NMC *Code* (2018b) states:

10.3: exercise professional accountability in ensuring the safe administration of medicines to those receiving care.

Although the nurse administering the IV medication should have checked the calculation before administering the medication, nursing associates are also accountable for their actions in relation to safe drug administration, so it is important that both individuals involved report the incident, ensure the patient is stable and learn from this drug error.

Case study 12 Lydia (page 25)

1. Calculate how much nystatin is needed per dose.
   100,000 units per ml ∴ **1ml of nystatin x 4 times a day**

2. Why does Lydia also need to be treated for thrush?

   Both Lydia and Myles have got thrush as it has been transmitted via the breast-feeding process. This yeast infection is the reason why Lydia is finding feeding painful and why Myles is unsettled, uncomfortable and not feeding as well. Unless both are treated successfully, the problem will not resolve. Advice around ensuring that medication is continued after lesions disappear (10 days for Lydia and 48 hours for Myles) is crucial for the treatment to be effective.

3. If 2 per cent of the cream contains miconazole, how many mg is there in a 20mg tube?
   $2 \div 100 \times 20 =$ **0.4mg miconazole in 20mg tube**

4. Look up paroxetine and sertraline in the BNF. What is the advice around using this medication in pregnancy? Why was her antidepressant medication swapped at the start of her pregnancy?

   There is an increased risk of congenital issues with paroxetine as opposed to other Selective Serotonin Reuptake Inhibitors (SSRIs) such as sertraline, so she was swapped to a lower risk medication.

5. Look up sertraline in LactMed: **https://toxnet.nlm.nih.gov/newtoxnet/lactmed.htm.** What is the advice about using sertraline when breastfeeding?

   Although sertraline can pass through the breast milk barrier, the levels of the drug are very low. Sertraline is considered one of the safer antidepressant options for breastfeeding women. As the risk of medication passing through the breast milk is less than through the placenta, women are usually advised to remain on the antidepressant they were on during pregnancy while they breastfeed.

6. Are there benefits to Lydia continuing to breastfeed? If so, what are they?
   United Nations International Children's Emergency Fund (2019) outline a range of breastfeeding benefits including:

- Babies have reduced risk of developing certain infections and conditions such as heart disease and asthma.
- Mothers have a reduced risk of developing ovarian or breast cancer.
- It is free and helps build a bond between mother and baby.

7. Using the Royal College of Paediatrics and Child Health (RCPCH) growth chart, calculate which centile Myles was for his weight, height and head circumference two weeks ago.

    He was on the 2nd centile for weight, height and head circumference.

8. Calculate which centile Myles is on today for his weight, height and head circumference. What does this indicate?

    Today, he is on the 0.4th centile for weight, height and head circumference. This indicates that he has not adequately put on weight in the last two weeks, as Lydia had thought. This needs closely monitoring to prevent further deterioration.

Case study 13: Maternity survey (page XX)

1. There has been a positive upward trend since 2017 in people receiving no delay in their discharge from hospital. What is this increase expressed as a percentage?
    62% − 55% = 7%

2. $^3/_4$ of respondents had been asked about their Mental health in the antenatal period, if 20,000 people responded to the questionnaire, how many had been asked about their Mental Health?
    75 ÷ 100 x 20,000 = 15,000 people

3. A fifth of respondents did not have a choice of where to deliver, how many people is this based on a respondent number of 20,000?
    1÷5 × 20,000 = 4,000

4. What is 102 per 1000 births as a percentage? What is 74 per 1000 births as a percentage? What is the difference between these figures as an indication of inequality pertaining to maternal re-admission?
    102 ÷ 1000 = 0.102 x 100 = 10.2%
    74 ÷ 1000 = 0.074 x 100 = 7.4%
    10.2% and 7.4% demonstrates greater re-admission numbers in black African and black Caribbean women who had given birth.

5. What is the difference in the number of Midwives between July 2021 and July 2022?
    26,556 − 26,041 = 515 less Midwives.

6. What is the difference in the number of births in England and Wales between 2021 and 2022?
    624,828 - 613,936 = 10,892 less births in 2022

7. On reflection what are the implications of a reduction in Midwife numbers and the inequalities in health care provision for different service users' groups?

    There is no sample answer to this question, but your reflection may allow you to consider inequalities in health care provision in other services and possible actions we can all take.

Further reading

The following sources are particularly recommended for further reading around the pharmacology of drugs, the pharmacokinetics and dynamics.

Department of Health (2017) Drug misuse and dependence. UK guidelines on clinical management. https://assets.publishing.service.gov.uk/government/uploads/system/uploads/attachment_data/file/673978/clinical_guidelines_2017.pdf

Neal, MJ (2020) *Medical Pharmacology at a Glance* (9th edn). Oxford: Wiley Blackwell.

NICE (2018) Dementia: assessment, management and support for people living with dementia and their carers. Recommendations | Dementia: assessment, management and support for people living with dementia and their carers | Guidance | NICE

Young, S and Pitcher, B (2016) *Medicines Management for Nurses at a Glance.* West Sussex: Wiley Blackwell.

Useful websites

BAPEN: www.bapen.org.uk/

The 'MUST' screening tool is available via the BAPEN website, as well as a range of BMI and weight-loss charts that are available to download.

BNF Online: https://bnf.nice.org.uk/

The BNF should be used as a reference to learn more about the indications, recommended doses and side effects of any prescribed medication.

LactMed: https://toxnet.nlm.nih.gov/newtoxnet/lactmed.htm

This website provides evidence-based information regarding whether certain medications are recommended during lactation and breastfeeding or not.

MHRA Drug-name confusion: www.gov.uk/drug-safety-update/drug-name-confusion-reminder-to-be-vigilant-for-potential-errors

This is a drug safety update reminding healthcare professionals to be vigilant for potential errors when dealing with medications that sound or look similar; examples are provided.

Royal College of Paediatrics and Child Health Growth Charts: www.rcpch.ac.uk/resources/uk-who-growth-charts-0-4-years

This provides a link to access the UK World Health Organization growth charts for children.

PHQ9 and GAD7 screening tool (page 31)

www.england.nhs.uk/wp-content/uploads/2018/06/iapt-manual-resources-v2.pdf

A screening tool for anxiety and depression, commonly used in clinical settings.

Electronic Medicines Compendium: www.medicines.org.uk/emc

This website provides information on pharmacodynamics and kinetics.

Resus Council: www.resus.org.uk/

This website provides clinical guidelines and algorithms for the treatment of a range of emergency situations. It includes a framework for the ABCDE assessment and algorithm for anaphylaxis, both discussed within this chapter.

Side Effects of Medicines FAQs: www.gov.uk/government/organisations/medicines-and-healthcare-products-regulatory-agency

Regulatory medicines body that produces regular safety updates to minimise drug errors, interactions or adverse effects.

World Health Organization Pain Ladder: www.who.int/cancer/palliative/painladder/en/

This is a standardised stepped approach to pain management utilised regularly in practice.

Glossary

absorption   the movement of a drug from the site of administration to the bloodstream.

absorption rate   the time from when the medicine is administered to its entry into the bloodstream.

accountability   the explanation of your actions or omissions to individuals to whom you owe a duty.

accountable officer   someone denoted within the organisation with specific responsibility for all aspects of controlled drug management.

accumulation   gradual build-up of a substance.

active transport   the movement of molecular substances across a cell membrane requiring energy.

acute pain   short duration unpleasant sensation provoked by disease or injury.

acute psychotic episode   the perception or interpretation of reality in an altered way; may include hallucinations and delusions.

adjuvants   substance that accelerates, prolongs or enhances a treatment; medicine licenced for other purposes but utilised for pain management due to additional analgesic effect.

administration   the giving of a medication to a patient while you observe them taking it or assisting them with this process.

adverse drug reaction (ADR)   any unwanted or harmful reaction that occurs after the administration of a medicine, which has occurred directly because of the drug.

advocate   a person who makes a decision or puts a case on someone else's behalf.

aetiology   the cause of disease.

affective disorder   set of mental health disorders that alter the mood.

affinity   the ability or likelihood of a medicine to bind to its target.

agonist   a substance whose molecular structure is similar in shape to the body's natural chemical, binds to a receptor and initiates a physiological response.

anaphylaxis   severe and potentially life-threatening response to a trigger.

antagonist   a substance whose molecular structure is similar to the body's natural chemical, binds to the receptor and inhibits a physiological response.

antibiotic guardian   campaign led by Public Health England urging prescribers and service user to take action to slow antibiotic resistance.

antimicrobial resistance   when microorganisms adapt and mutate in ways that render medications used to cure the infections they cause ineffective.

antimicrobial stewardship   systematic effort to educate prescribers and service users to follow evidence-based prescribing to reduce antimicrobial overuse and resistance.

antimotility   medications that slow down bowel peristalsis or movement.

anxiety   a feeling of worry, nervousness or unease about something with an uncertain outcome.

apoptosis   the rapid and irreversible process of programmed death of cells.

atoms   the smallest unit of matter.

bioavailability   the proportion of a medicine that enters the circulation and is able to have an active effect.

biotransformation   the alteration of a substance into components or metabolites.

blood–brain barrier   highly selective semi-permeable membrane that prevents some substances crossing into the fluid of the nervous system.

Body Mass Index (BMI)   an approximate measure of ideal weight calculated by dividing a person's weight in kilograms by the square of their height in metres.

capacity   having the ability to make one's own decisions.

carcinogenesis   a process which initiates the formation of a cancer.

Care Quality Commission (CQC)   independent regulator of all health and social care in England.

carrier proteins   substance that transport ions and small molecules across the cell membrane.

cell   the most basic structural, functional and biological unit of living organisms.

cerebral cortex   outer layer of the cerebrum composed of grey matter which plays an important role in consciousness.

chemical digestion   use of enzymes to break down gut contents, digesting proteins into smaller amino acids and fats into triglycerides to prepare for absorption.

chemical name   the chemical composition and molecular structure of a medicine.

chronic pain   unpleasant sensation of lengthy duration – more than three months – which outlasts the usual healing process.

chime   pulpy acidic fluid consisting of gastric liquids and partly digested food.

clinical audit   the collation and examination of information about care within your organisation to allow improvement.

clinical governance   activities that help sustain and improve high standards of patient care.

clinical management plan (CMP)   an agreed defined plan of treatment that sets legal boundaries for medication prescribing.

competence   the ability to do something successfully within boundaries of skill acquisition and knowledge.

concentration gradient   the difference in amount of substance in a defined space on each side of a membrane.

concordance   an agreement reached between healthcare professionals and service users regarding medicines regimens.

consent   permission for something to happen.

contraindication   a reason to withhold a medicine due to the harm it could cause.

controlled drugs (CDs)   medicines subject to additional restrictions and controls on their use.

covert   administration of medication to individuals who are unable to give informed consent to treatment and who refuse medication when they are openly offered.

critical and major incidents   urgent and significant threat to life that requires multiple resources to manage.

critical medications   medications that require strict adherence to dosage times to reduce the potential for severely debilitating symptoms to reoccur for service users.

dementia   overall term for syndrome characterised by symptoms, including cognitive decline.

depot   medication delivered as a reservoir of drug allowing slow, sustained release.

depression   feelings of severe despondency and dejection.

deprivation of liberty safeguards (DoLS)   ensuring that people are looked after in a way that does not take advantage of those whose freedom is restricted.

dispensing   the provision of medication for the patient to take away.

distribution   how the medicine is spread around the body.

drug dependence   the adaption of the body to the repeated exposure to a medicine, which means that the body only functions normally in the presence of that medicine.

drug interaction   an effect or action as a result of administration of a drug at the same time as another medicine or food substance.

drug misuse   the use of a substance for a purpose not consistent with legal or medical guidelines.

duration of action   the time the medicine continues to produce its therapeutic, diagnostic or preventative effect.

duty of candour   open culture allowing honest provision of information and apologies if necessary.

electron   subatomic particle with a negative electrical charge.

enteral   medicine administration involving the oesophagus, stomach and small and large intestines.

enzyme inhibitors   substance that prevents the body's enzymes from promoting or accelerating normal biochemical reactions.

excretion   the process of elimination or expelling waste from the body.

extracellular   located outside the cell membrane.

facilitated diffusion   the use of carrier proteins to move molecules across the cell membrane from the area of high to low concentration.

fingertip unit (FTU)   a dosage measure for creams and ointments.

first pass metabolism   the reduction in the concentration of a medicine into the systemic circulation of a drug administered orally because of metabolism by the liver.

formulary   a list of medications.

Fraser guidelines relate to one of the Lords responsible for the judgement of the Gillick court case who went on to address the specific issue of contraceptive advice and treatment.

gate control theory of pain put forward by Melzack and Wall in 1965 as an explanation as to how pain can be prevented from travelling to the central nervous system to reduce painful stimulus.

general sales list medicines (GSLs) products with the lowest level of control over their sale and supply; they can be sold from any lockable outlet.

generic name indicates the active ingredient of the medicine.

genomics investigation of molecular structure, function, evolution and mapping of chromosomes.

Gillick competence a term used in English law to decide whether a child under 16 can consent to medical treatment.

half-life the time taken for the plasma concentration of the medicine to fall by half of its original value.

herd immunity a population is protected from a disease after vaccination by stopping the microorganism responsible for the infection being transmitted between people.

homeostasis the maintenance of a stable environment or equilibrium by physiological processes.

hypersensitive an extreme sensitivity to an antigen initiating an immune response.

iatrogenic describes illness caused by medical treatment.

implied consent consent which is not expressly granted but implicitly granted by action.

independent prescribers can prescribe any licensed medicine and unlicensed medicines within their formulary.

inflammation body's defence mechanism at the site of injury or trauma; classic signs include redness, warmth, pain and swelling derived from increased vascular permeability to allow pathogens to be destroyed and tissue repaired.

informed consent permission granted for something to happen in full knowledge of possible risks and benefits.

inhaler a metred dose device that allows delivery of medicines to the respiratory system.

interphase when the cell grows and undertakes its normal activities.

interstitial space spaces between tissues or parts of organs.

intracellular located within the cell membrane.

ion charged atom with an unequal number of electrons and protons.

ion channels selective pores in the membrane of the cell that allow the transfer of ions.

labelling attached specific required information to medication to ensure safety.

lasting power of attorney (LPA) a legal document recognising that a person is able to make decisions on someone's behalf.

laxative medicine that stimulates or facilitates evacuation of the bowels.

liberty protection safeguards replacement of DoLS as the system of protection for those lawfully deprived of their liberty.

lymphocytes white blood cells that respond to and destroy specific 'non-self' invaders.

Malnutrition Universal Screening Tools' ('MUST') a five-step screening tool to identify adults who are malnourished, at risk of malnutrition or obese; includes management guidelines.

margin of safety range of safety between an effective dose and a lethal one.

mechanical digestion the breakdown of food substances through the action of accessory organs, including salivary glands, the tongue and teeth.

medical emergency acute injury or illness that poses an immediate risk to a person's life or long-term health.

metabolism a whole range of chemical reactions that allow the breaking down of substances.

metric system system of weights and measurements that allows an International system of units used in almost all countries.

mitigate against to take measures to alleviate or moderate harm; to lessen the force or intensity of outcome of risk event.

mitotic phase when replicated chromosomes are separated into two new nuclei in daughter cells.

neurogenic inflammation physiological process by which substances are released directly from the nerve to initiate a protective response.

NHS Healthy Weight Calculator a chart to indicate whether a person is a healthy weight for their height.

National Institute for Health and Care Excellence (NICE) independent organisation responsible for promoting and instigating improvement and excellence in the health and social care system.

near-miss an event that might have resulted in harm but, due to a timely intervention by healthcare providers or the patient or their family, did not result in injury.

nebuliser device that converts medicine into a fine spray for inhalation.

never event serious, largely preventable patient safety incident that should not occur if healthcare providers have implemented national guidance.

nociceptive relating to the perception or sensation of pain.

non-medical prescribers a recognised practitioner who is not a doctor but who is able to select appropriate medication for a service user.

off-licence product is being used for a purpose for which it does not have a licence.

one-stop dispensing combining inpatient and discharge dispensing into one single supply.

onset of action the time taken for the medicine to start working once administered.

opiates a medicine derived from or related to the opium used to sedate and treat pain.

parenteral medicines taken into the body in a manner other than through the digestive canal.

passive diffusion the movement of molecular substances across a cell membrane without the requirement for any energy or effort.

pathogens infective agents such as bacteria, virus, fungus and parasites which can cause disease.

pathophysiology the study of the disordered physiological processes associated with disease or injury.

palliative care the treatment, care and support for people with life-limiting illness.

patient group directions (PGDs) allow certain, identified professional groups to administer drugs in line with strict criteria and instructions laid out in the directive to groups of individuals clearly defined in the document.

patient-specific direction medicine is prescribed for a specific individual as a written instruction.

peak concentration the highest concentration of the medicine in the blood or target organ after administration.

peristalsis the contraction and relaxation of gut muscles to aid movement through the gastrointestinal tract.

personal protective equipment (PPE) clothing and equipment that protects the wearer against health and safety risks at work.

phagocytes type of white blood cells that engulf and destroy invading organisms.

pharmacist specialist, expert practitioner with knowledge, skill and precision to safely prepare and dispense medications.

pharmacy medicines (P-medicines) drugs sold by a pharmacist or under the supervision of a pharmacist from a registered pharmacy premises.

pharmacodynamics the biochemical effects of the medicines and their mechanisms of action or drug effect.

pharmacogenomics the study that explores unique differences to medicines based on genetic make-up.

pharmacokinetics explaining the absorption, distribution, metabolism and excretion of medicines.

pharmacotherapeutics the use of medicines to prevent and treat conditions.

pharmacovigilance the monitoring of medicines to identify and evaluate unknown and unwanted effects.

pinocytosis the engulfing of a liquid by the budding of small vesicles from the cell membrane.

placebo effect an individual's belief in the value of the medicine produces a beneficial effect which cannot be attributed to the substance.

placenta organ attached to the wall of the uterus and foetus's umbilical cord which supplies nutrients and oxygen, and removes waste from the foetal blood supply.

polypharmacy the prescribing of more than four different medicines to one individual.

portal an additional network of vessels between arterial and venous circulation which do not drain into the heart; the portal vein brings nutrient-rich blood to the liver from the gastrointestinal tract.

prescribing the selection of the appropriate medication by a recognised practitioner.

prescription only medicines (POMs)   drugs sold or supplied when there is a prescription written which authorises the transaction.

prophylactic   the administration of a medicine to prevent disease.

proprietary name   the trade name of a drug that can only be used by the patent owner.

prostaglandins   a group of lipids made at the site of tissue damage which control the immune response.

proton   subatomic particle with a positive electrical charge.

pruritis   unpleasant itching sensation of the skin.

pyrexia   raised body temperature.

pyrogens   a substance, usually a bacterium, which produces a high body temperature or fever when introduced into the bloodstream.

receptors   a region of tissue on the cell membrane which responds specifically to the body's natural chemicals, transmitter substances, mediators or hormones.

recommended International Nonproprietary Name (rINN)   unique, internationally recognised name of a medicine which identifies the active pharmaceutical ingredient.

responsibility   the sense of ownership for the quality of your actions.

'rights'   of medicine administration are several steps taken to minimise the potential for error.

risk management   allows individual risk events to be understood and managed proactively.

safety critical medicines   medicines that carry a high risk of harm.

schedules and classes   schedule is a list or inventory in a formal document. Medicines are divided into the five schedules or lists dependent on their potential for harm and abuse. The class A/B/C dictates the penalty in law associated with the production, supply and possession of these drugs.

secure stationery   denotes a legal document with tight controls to allow regulation of the ordering of, storage, use and disposal.

sepsis   potentially life-threatening condition as a result of body's response to an infection.

serious adverse events   any undesirable or unintended sign or symptom of a disease associated with treatment.

signs   the objective evidence of disease.

social prescribing   a non-pharmacological treatment where GPs and other healthcare professionals can refer people to 'activities' or services in their community instead of offering only medical solutions.

spacer   a device that attaches to an inhaler and holds the medication until it can be breathed in.

specificity   the level of selectivity to one receptor.

standard operating procedures (SOPs)   a document explaining the procedures, accountability and responsibilities of employers when dealing with controlled drugs.

suffixes   common endings that are used to denote medicines with similar pharmaceutical characteristics or mechanisms of action.

supplementary prescribing   a voluntary partnership between the patient, a non-medical prescriber and an independent prescriber who must be a doctor or a dentist.

supply   the giving of medicines to a service user for them to take away and take over a specified period and in a certain way.

symptoms   subjective description of disease processes.

teratogenesis   the process by which congenital foetal abnormalities occur.

thalamus   grey matter located between the cerebral hemispheres which relays sensory information.

therapeutic   administration of a medicine to treat a condition, control the disease progression or reduce unpleasant symptoms.

therapeutic index   the relationship between a medicine's desired effect and the adverse effects.

tolerance   the alteration of the effect of a substance after continued subjection/use.

topically   medicine administered to a target site of the body surface.

tort law   within common law jurisdiction, it is a civil wrong that causes the claimant to suffer loss or harm.

unlicensed   product does not hold a marketing authorisation, administered and monitored by the Medicines and Healthcare Products Regulatory Agency.

urticarial   raised rash caused by a reaction to a substance.

vaccine hesitancy   a reluctance of an adult or child to have a vaccine administered despite the availability of vaccination services.

vicarious liability   this legal principle protects employees from individual litigation.

yellow card   produced by the MHRA to allow the reporting of suspected adverse drug reactions.

References

Academy of Medical Colleges (2022) *Statement on the Initial Antimicrobial Treatment of Sepsis V2.0.* Available at: https://www.aomrc.org.uk/reports-guidance/statement-on-the-initial-antimicrobial-treatment-of-sepsis-v2-0/

Ancona, A., Petito, C., Iavarone, I., Petito, V., Galasso, L., Leonetti, A., Turchini, L., Belella, D., Ferrarrese, D., Addolorato, G., Armuzzi, A., Gasbarrini, A. and Scaldaferri, F. (2021) The gut–brain axis in irritable bowel syndrome and inflammatory bowel disease. *Digestive and Liver Disease*, 53(3): 298–305. Available at: https://www-sciencedirect-com.salford.idm.oclc.org/science/article/pii/S159086582031046X

Ashelford, S., Raynsford, J. and Taylor, V. (2024) *Pathophysiology and Pharmacology in Nursing* (3rd edn). London: SAGE.

Audit Commission (2001) *A Spoonful of Sugar: Medicines Management in NHS Hospitals.* London: Audit Commission. Available at: www.eprescribingtoolkit.com/wp-content/uploads/2013/11/nrspoonfulsugar1.pdf (accessed 19 October 2022).

British Association for Parental and Enteral Nutrition (BAPEN) (2011) *Introducing 'MUST'.* Available at: www.bapen.org.uk/screening-and-must/must/introducing-must (accessed 16 April 2020).

British National Formulary (BNF) (2023) London: BMJ Group/Pharmaceutical Press. Available at: www.bnf.org/bnf/

CQC (2015) *Regulation 20: Duty of Candour.* Available at: https://www.cqc.org.uk/guidance-providers/all-services/regulation-20-duty-candour (accessed 19 October 2022).

CQC (2019) *2018 Adult Inpatient Survey: Statistics Released.* Available at: www.cqc.org.uk/sites/default/files/20190620_ip18_statisticalrelease.pdf

Care Quality Commission (2022a) *The Safer Management of Controlled Drugs: Annual Report 2021.* Available at: https://www.cqc.org.uk/publication/safer-management-controlled-drugs (accessed 18 October 2022).

Care Quality Commission (2022b) *Covert Administering of Medicines.* Available at: https://www.cqc.org.uk/guidance-providers/adult-social-care/covert-administration-medicines (accessed 19 October 2022).

CQC (2022c) *Maternity Survey.* Available at: https://www.cqc.org.uk/publication/surveys/maternity-survey-2022

Cook, N., et al. (2021) *Essentials of Anatomy and Physiology* (2nd edn). London: SAGE.

DHSS (Department of Health and Social Care) (2019a) *Advancing Our Health: Prevention in the 2020s – Consultation Document.* Available at: www.gov.uk/government/consultations/advancing-our-health-prevention-in-the-2020s/advancing-our-health-prevention-in-the-2020s-consultation-document

DHSS (2019b) *UK 20-year Vision for Antimicrobial Resistance.* Available at: www.gov.uk/government/publications/uk-20-year-vision-for-antimicrobial-resistance

European Council. *Directive 2004/27/EC of the European Parliament and Council of 31 March 2004 amending Directive 2001/83/EC on the Community Code Relating to Medicinal Products for Human Use.* Available at: https://eur-lex.europa.eu/legal-content/EN/TXT/?uri=CELEX:32004L0027 (accessed 19 October 2022).

European Parliamentary Research Service (2015) *Medicinal Products in the European Union*. Available at: https://www.europarl.europa.eu/RegData/etudes/IDAN/2015/554174/EPR-S_IDA(2015)554174_EN.pdf (accessed 18 October 2022).

EMC (Electronic Medicines Compendium) (n.d.) Available at: www.medicines.org.uk/emc

Gaskin, S. (2019) *Behavioral Neuroscience: Essentials and beyond*. Thousand Oaks, CA: SAGE.

Gates, B., Fearns, D. and Welch, J. (2015) *Learning Disability Nursing at a Glance*. Chichester: John Wiley & Sons. Available at: http://ebookcentral.proquest.com/lib/uocuk/detail.action?docID=1895473

Gillick vs. West Norfolk and Wisbech Area Health Authority (1985) Available at: https://ministryofethics.co.uk/index.php?p=7&q=2 (accessed 20 October 2022).

Global Initiative for Asthma (2019) *A Pocket Guide for Health Professionals*. Available at: https://ginasthma.org/wp-content/uploads/2019/04/GINA-2019-main-Pocket-Guide-wms.pdf

HEE (Health Education England) (2016) Nursing associate curriculum framework. Available at: www.hee.nhs.uk/news-blogs-events/news/nursing-associate-curriculum-framework (accessed 20 September 2019).

HEE (2017) *Advisory Guidance: Administration of Medicines by Nursing Associates*. Available at: www.hee.nhs.uk/sites/default/files/documents/Advisory%20guidance%20-%20adminis tration%20of%20medicines%20by%20nursing%20associates.pdf (accessed 19 October 2022).

HMSO (1968) *Medicines Act 1968*. London: HMSO. Available at: https://www.legislation.gov.uk/ukpga/1968/67 (accessed 20 October 2022).

HMSO (1971) *Misuse of Drugs Act 1971*. London: HMSO. Available at: https://www.legislation.gov.uk/ukpga/1971/38 (accessed 20 October 2022).

HMSO (1974) *Health and Safety at Work Act 1974*. Available at: www.hse.gov.uk/legislation/hswa.htm (accessed 20 October 2022).

HMSO (1983) *Mental Health Act 1983*. London: HMSO. Available at: www.legislation.gov.uk/ukpga/1983/20/contents/enacted (accessed 20 October 2022).

HMSO (1995) *Disability Discrimination Act 1995*. London: HMSO. Available at: www.legislation.gov.uk/ukpga/1995/50/contents (accessed 20 October 2022).

HMSO (2001) *Misuse of Drugs Regulations 2001*. London: HMSO. Available at: www.legislation.gov.uk/uksi/2001/3998/contents/made (accessed 20 October 2022).

HMSO (2002) *The Nursing and Midwifery Order 2001*. London: HMSO. Available at: www.legislation.gov.uk/uksi/2002/253/contents/made (accessed 20 October 2022).

HMSO (2004) *Children's Act 2004*. London: HMSO. Available at: www.legislation.gov.uk/ukpga/2004/31/contents/enacted (accessed 20 October 2022).

HMSO (2005) *Mental Capacity Act 2005*. London: HMSO. Available at: www.legislation.gov.uk/ukpga/2005/9/contents/enacted (accessed 19 October 2022).

HMSO (2006) *Health Act 2006*. London: HMSO. Available at: www.legislation.gov.uk/ukpga/2006/28/contents/enacted (accessed 20 October 2022).

HMSO (2007a) *Mental Health Act (Amendment Bill)*. London: HMSO. Available at: www.legislation.gov.uk/ukpga/2007/12/contents (accessed 19 October 2022).

HMSO (2009) *Health Act 2009*. London: HMSO. Available at: https://www.legislation.gov.uk/ukpga/2009/21/contents (accessed 18 October 2022).

HMSO (2010) *Equality Act*. London: HMSO. Available at: www.legislation.gov.uk/ukpga/2010/15/contents (accessed 20 October 2022).

HMSO (2012) *Human Medicines Regulations 2012*. London: HMSO. Available at: www.legislation.gov.uk/uksi/2012/1916/pdfs/uksi_20121916_en.pdf (accessed 20 October 2022).

HMSO (2013) *Controlled Drugs (Supervision of Management and Use) Regulations*. London: HMSO. Available at: https://www.legislation.gov.uk/uksi/2013/373/contents/made (accessed 18 October 2022).

HMSO (2014a) *Care Act 2014*. London: HMSO. Available at: www.legislation.gov.uk/ukpga/2014/23/contents/enacted (accessed 20 October 2022).

HMSO (2014b) *The Health and Social Care Act 2008 (Regulated Activities) Regulations 2014*. Available at: www.legislation.gov.uk/ukdsi/2014/9780111117613/contents (accessed 20 October 2022).

HMSO (2018) *General Data Protection Act 2018*. London: HMSO. Available at: www.legislation.gov.uk/ukpga/2018/12/contents/enacted (accessed 20 October 2022).

HMSO (2019) *Mental Capacity (Amendment) Bill*. London: HMSO. Available at: www.gov.uk/government/publications/mental-capacity-amendment-bill-easy-read (accessed 19 October 2022).

HMSO (2020) *The Human Medicines (Coronavirus and Influenza) (Amendment) Regulations 2020*. Available at: https://www.legislation.gov.uk/uksi/2020/1125/contents/made

HMSO (2021) *The Human Medicines (Coronavirus and Influenza) (Amendment) Regulations 2021*. Available at: https://www.legislation.gov.uk/uksi/2022/350/note/made

Home Office Circular (2018) *Rescheduling of Cannabis-Based Products for Medicinal Use in Humans*. Available at: https://www.gov.uk/government/publications/circular-0182018-rescheduling-of-cannabis-based-products-for-medicinal-use-in-humans (accessed 20 October 2022).

House of Lords Select Committee on Science and Technology (2000) *Sixth Report*. Available at: https://publications.parliament.uk/pa/ld199900/ldselect/ldsctech/123/12301.htm

HSMO (2007) *Safeguarding Patients. The Government's Response to the Recommendations of the Shipman Inquiry's Fifth Report and to the Recommendations of the Ayling, Neale and Kerr/Haslam Inquiries*. Available at: https://assets.publishing.service.gov.uk/government/uploads/system/uploads/attachment_data/file/228872/7015.pdf (accessed 20 October 2022).

HSMO (2021) *The National Health Service (Performers Lists, Coronavirus) (England) Amendment Regulations 2021*. Available at: https://www.legislation.gov.uk/uksi/2021/30/regulation/1/made

Independent Committee on Toxicity of chemicals in food, consumer products and the environment (COT) (2017) *Statement on Heat Not Burn Tobacco Products*. Available at: https://cot.food.gov.uk/cotstatements/cotstatementsyrs/cot-statements-2017/statement-on-heat-not-burn-tobacco-products (accessed 16 April 2020).

Institute for Apprenticeships and Technical Education (2022). *Nursing Associate Standard STO827*. Available at: https://www.instituteforapprrenticeships.org/apprenticeship-standards/nursing-associate-nmc-2018-v1-1

Massachusetts Institute of Technology. (2021) News bulletin. Available at: https://news.mit.edu/2021/monoclonal-drug-delivery-capsule-0830

Medicines and Healthcare products Regulatory Agency [MHRA] (2022) *About Us*. Available at: https://www.gov.uk/government/organisations/medicines-and-healthcare-products-regulatory-agency/about

Melzack, R. and Wall, P. D. (1965) Pain mechanism: A new theory. *Science*, 150: 971–979.

Mersey Care Clinical Guidelines (2017) *Clinical Guidelines/Formulary Document: Psychosis and Schizophrenia*. Available at: www.merseycare.nhs.uk/media/3319/psychosis-and-schizophrenia-2017-final.pdf

National Institute for Health and Care Excellence (2014) *Behaviour Change: Individual Approaches. Public Health Guidance [PH49]*. Available at: https://www.nice.org.uk/guidance/ph49/chapter/glossary (accessed 25 October 2022).

NICE (2015a) *Antimicrobial Stewardship: Systems and Antimicrobial Stewardship: Systems and Processes for Effective Antimicrobial Medicine Use*. Available at: www.nice.org.uk/guidance/ng15/resources/antimicrobial-stewardship-systems-and-processes-for-effective-antimicrobial-medicine-use-pdf-1837273110469

References

NICE (2015b) *Clostridium Difficile Infection: Risk with Broad Spectrum Antiobiotics.* Available at: www.nice.org.uk/advice/esmpb1/chapter/key-points-from-the-evidence

NICE (2015c) *Medicines Optimisation: The Safe and Effective Use of Medicines to Enable the Best Possible Outcomes.* Available at: www.nice.org.uk/guidance/ng5 (accessed 19 October 2022).

NICE (2017a) *Asthma: Diagnosis, Monitoring and Chronic Asthma Management.* Available at: www.nice.org.uk/guidance/ng80

NICE (2017b) *Multimorbidity and Polypharmacy.* Available at: www.nice.org.uk/advice/ktt18/resources/multimorbidity-and-polypharmacy-pdf-58757959453381

NICE (2018) *Donepezil, Galantamine, Rivastigmine and Memantine for the Treatment of Alzheimer's Disease (TA217).* Available at: www.nice.org.uk/search?q=donepezil

National Institute for Health and Care Excellence (2019a) *Giving Medicine Covertly.* Available at: https://www.nice.org.uk/media/default/about/nice-communities/social-care/quick-guides/giving-medicines-covertly-quick-guide.pdf (accessed 19 October 2022).

NICE (2019b) *Generalised Anxiety Disorder and Panic Disorder in Adults: Management. Clinical Guidance (CG113).* Available at: www.nice.org.uk/guidance/cg113

NICE (2019c) *Depression in Adults: Recognition and Management (CG90).* Available at: www.nice.org.uk/search?q=Depression

NICE (2019d) *Antimicrobial Prescribing Guidelines.* Available at: www.nice.org.uk/about/what-we-do/our-programmes/nice-guidance/antimicrobial-prescribing-guidelines

National Institute for Health and Care Excellence (2019e) *Acute Kidney Injury: Prevention, Detection and Management.* Available at: https://www.nice.org.uk/guidance/ng148

National Institute for Health and Care Excellence (2020) *Anaphylaxis: Assessment and Referral after Emergency Treatment.* Available at: https://www.nice.org.uk/guidance/cg134 (accessed 18 October 2023).

National Institute for Health and Care Excellence (2021) *Cannabis-based Medicinal Products.* Available at: https://www.nice.org.uk/guidance/ng144/resources/cannabisbased-medicinal-products-clarification-of-guidance-march-2021-9070302205 (accessed 18 October 2022).

National Institute for Health and Care Excellence (2022) *Obesity: Identification, Assessment and Management [CG189].* Available at: https://www.nice.org.uk/guidance/cg189

NHS England (2018) *Mental Health Choice Guidance.* Available at: www.england.nhs.uk/2014/12/mh-choice-guidance/

NHS England (2019b) *The NHS Longterm Plan.* Available at: www.longtermplan.nhs.uk/wp-content/uploads/2019/01/the-nhs-long-term-plan-summary.pdf

NHS England (2021) *National Patient Safety Incident Reports Up to June 2021.* Available at: https://www.england.nhs.uk/publication/national-patient-safety-incident-reports-up-to-june-2021/

NHS Improvement (2019) *NRLS National Patient Safety Incident Reports: Commentary.* Available at: https://improvement.nhs.uk/documents/5065/NAPSIR_commentary_March_2019_Final.pdf

NHS Specialist Pharmacy Service (2018) *Medicines Matters: A Guide to Mechanisms for the Prescribing, Supply and Administration of Medicines (In England).* Available at: https://www.sps.nhs.uk/articles/medicines-mattersa-guide-to-mechanisms-for-the-prescribing-supply-and-administration-of-medicines-in-england/ (accessed 20 October 2022).

Normansell, R., Kew, K. M., Stovold, E., Mathioudakis, A. and Dennett, E. (2017) Interventions to improve inhaler technique and adherence to inhaled corticosteroids in children with asthma. *Paediatric Respiratory Reviews.* Available at: https://doi.org/10.1016/j.prrv.2017.03.014

NMC (Nursing and Midwifery Counci) (2018a) *Standards of Proficiency for Nursing Associates*. London: NMC. Available at: www.nmc.org.uk/globalassets/sitedocuments/education-standards/nursing-associates-proficiency-standards.pdf (accessed 14 April 2020).

NMC (2018b) *The Code: Professional Standards of Practice and Behaviour for Nurses, Midwives and Nursing Associates*. London: NMC. Available at: www.nmc.org.uk/globalassets/sitedocuments/nmc-publications/nmc-code.pdf (accessed 19 October 2022).

Nursing and Midwifery Council (2022) *Guidance on the Professional Duty of Candour*. London: NMC. Available at: https://www.nmc.org.uk/standards/guidance/the-professional-duty-of-candour/ (accessed 19 October 2022).

Nutbeam, T. and Daniels, R. on behalf of the UK Sepsis Trust (2019) *What Is Sepsis?* Available at: sepsistrust.org/professional-resources/clinical (accessed 16 December 2019).

PresQUIPP (2022) *Bulletin 269: Care Homes – Covert Administration*. Available at: https://www.prescqipp.info/our-resources/bulletins/bulletin-269-care-homes-covert-administration/ (accessed 19 October 2022).

PHE (Public Health England) (2017) *Health Matters: Obesity and the Food Environment*. Available at: www.gov.uk/government/publications/health-matters-obesity-and-the-food-environment/health-matters-obesity-and-the-food-environment (accessed 16 April 2020).

PHE (2019) *Turning the Tide on Tobacco: Smoking in England Hits a New Low*. Available at: https://publichealthmatters.blog.gov.uk/2018/07/03/turning-the-tide-on-tobacco-smoking-in-england-hits-a-new-low/ (accessed 16 April 2020).

Quick, J. D. and Larson, H. (2018) The vaccine-autism myth started 20 years ago. *TIME*. Available at: https://time.com/5175704/andrew-wakefield-vaccine-autism/

Resuscitation Council (UK) (2021a) *Resuscitation Guidelines 2021*. Available at: https://www.resus.org.uk/library/2021-resuscitation-guidelines

Resuscitation Council (UK) (2021b) *Emergency Treatment of Anaphylactic Reactions: Guidelines for Healthcare Providers*. Available at: https://www.resus.org.uk/library/additional-guidance/guidance-anaphylaxis/emergency-treatment (accessed 19 October 2022).

Royal College of Physicians (2017) *National Early Warning Score (NEWS) 2. Standardizing the Assessment of Acute-Illness Severity in the NHS*. Available at: www.rcplondon.ac.uk/projects/outputs/national-early-warning-score-news-2

Royal College of Psychiatrists (2022) *Cannabis and Mental Health*. Available at: https://www.rcpsych.ac.uk/mental-health/parents-and-young-people/young-people/cannabis-and-mental-health-information-for-young-people (accessed 18 October 2022).

RPS (Royal Pharmaceutical Society) (2013) *Medicines Optimisation: Helping Patients to Make the Most of Medicines*. Available at: www.rpharms.com/Portals/0/RPS%20document%20library/Open%20access/Policy/helping-patients-make-the-most-of-their-medicines.pdf

Royal Pharmaceutical Society (2023) *Professional Guidance on the Administration of Medicines in Healthcare Settings*. Available at: https://www.rpharms.com/Portals/0/RPS%20document%20library/Open%20access/Professional%20standards/SSHM%20and%20Admin/Admin%20of%20Meds%20prof%20guidance.pdf?ver=2019-01-23-145026-567

Scally, G. and Donaldson, L. G. (1998) A framework for the analysis of risk and safety in medicines. *BMJ*, 317: 61–65.

Tortora, G. and Derrikson, B. (2018) *Introduction to the Human Body* (11th edn). Hoboken: John Wiley & Sons.

United Nations International Children's Emergency Fund (2019) *The Best Start to Life*. Available at: www.unicef.org/programme/breastfeeding/ (accessed 16 April 2020).

WHO (World Health Organization) (1986) *Cancer Pain Ladder for Adults*. Available at: www.who.int/cancer/palliative/painladder/en/

References

WHO (2017a) *Antimicrobial Resistance.* Available at: www.who.int/antimicrobial-resistance/en/

WHO (2017b) *Medication without Harm: WHO Global Patient Safety Challenge.* Available at: https://apps.who.int/iris/bitstream/handle/10665/255263/WHO-HIS-SDS-2017.6-eng.pdf?sequence=1

WHO (2018b) *ICD-11 International Statistical Classification of Diseases and Related Health Problems (ICD).* Available at: www.who.int/classifications/icd/en/

WHO (2019) *Ten Threats to Global Health in 2019.* Available at: www.who.int/emergencies/ten-threats-to-global-health-in-2019

WHO (2020) *Global Report on the Epidemiology and Burden of Sepsis: Current Evidence, Identifying Gaps and Future Directions.* https://www.who.int/activities/improving-the-prevention-diagnosis-and-clinical-management-of-sepsis

Index

Absorption, 31–33, 47, 49, 54
  rate, 48, 64
Accountability, 2, 6, 9–10, 19, 20, 63
Accumulation, 33, 50, 54
Active transport, 28, 32, 47, 48 (figure)
Acute pain, 120, 121
Acute psychotic episodes, 123
Adenosine triphosphate (ATP), 47
Adjuvants, 37, 121
Administering liquids, 100–101
Administering tablets, 98–100
Administration, 8–10, 19, 35–36, 44–48. *See also* Safe
  medicines administration.
ADR. *See* Adverse drug reactions (ADR)
Adverse drug reactions (ADR),
  61, 73, 75
Advocate, 62, 132, 143
Aetiology, 36
Affective disorders, 123
Affinity, 49, 51
Ageing process, 35–36, 53
Agonists, 50, 51 (figure)
Airway, breathing, circulation, disability and exposure
  (ABCDE), 75
Alcohol consumption, 131
Antagonists, 51, 51 (figure)
Antibiotic guardian, 127
Antimicrobial resistance (AMR), 125–127
Antimicrobial stewardship, 126
Antimotility medications, 122
Anxiety, 2, 22, 35, 50, 52, 123
Apoptosis, 28
Artificial intelligence (AI), 130
Aspirin, 10, 49, 70, 121
Atoms, 48, 52
Awareness, 8, 19, 20, 122, 126

Bioavailability, 48
Biotransformation, 2, 49, 50
Blood–brain barrier, 49
Body Mass Index (BMI), 88, 90–92
Body mass index calculation, 89–92
Body systems, homoeostasis, 30 (figure)
British Association for Parenteral and Enteral
  Nutrition (BAPEN), 91, 95
British National Formulary (BNF), 10, 45, 82
Broad-spectrum antibiotics, 126

CAMs. *See* Complementary and alternative medicines
  (CAMs)

Capacity, 2, 20, 62
Carcinogenesis, 75
Carrier proteins, 47, 50, 52
Cells, 27–29, 32–33, 35
  structure, 27 (figure)
Cerebral cortex, 121
Chemical digestion, 32
Chemical name, 45, 64
Chronic pain, 64, 121
Chyme, 32
Circulatory system, 32, 34, 47, 54, 122
Clinical audit, 17
Clinical governance, 17–18
Clinical management plan (CMP), 19
Code of conduct, 6
Communication systems, 26, 28, 32, 40
Competence, 2, 17, 19–20, 62, 66, 83, 110, 138
Complementary and alternative medicines (CAMs),
  124–125
Concentration gradient, 32, 47
Concordance, 2, 7, 62, 123, 126
Consent, 61
Constipation, 32, 69, 122
Contraindication, 34, 66, 74
Controlled drugs (CDs), 11, 12–13
Controlled drugs (Supervision of management & use)
  Regulations 2013, 12
Conversion, 51, 85–88
Converting units, 139
Covert administration, 62–63
Critical and major incidents, 17
Critical medications, 64
Cyclooxygenase (COX) enzyme inhibitor, 51

Dangerous Drugs Act 1920, 12
Dementia, 36, 123
Depression, 37, 73, 123
Deprivation of liberty safeguards (DOLS), 62
Diagnostic systems, 129
Diamorphine, 121
Diarrhoea, 32, 37, 40, 54, 122
Digestive disorders, 33
Digestive system, 32
Disease process, 36–38
Dispensing, 19
Distribution, 2, 31, 34, 44, 49, 54
Drip rate calculation, 140
Drop rate, 103–104
Drug calculations, numeracy skills for
  administering liquids, 100–101

administering tablets, 98–100
application, 83 (table)–84 (table)
body mass index calculation, 89–92
calculations according to weight, 101–103
conversion, 85–88
drop rate, 103–104
flow rate, 104–105
fluid balance, 105–110, 106 (table)–109 (table)
imperial weight conversion, 88
infusion rates, 103
mathematical principles, 84–85
nearest whole number, 88–89
number fractions, 92–94
percentages, 94–96
ratios, 96–98
units of measurement, 85–88
Drug dependence, 127–128
Drug interaction, 73–75
Drug misuse, 127–128
Duration of action, 33, 50, 53
Duty of candour, 17, 66
Dyspepsia, 122

E-cigarettes, 130
Electrons, 48
Endocrine system, 28–29
Enteral feeds, 67
Environment, 16, 17, 27, 28, 32, 54, 66
Enzyme inhibitors, 46, 51
Excretion, 2, 32, 33, 45, 50, 74
Extracellular, 27

Facilitated diffusion, 47, 48 (figure)
Fingertip unit (FTU), 69
First pass metabolism, 33, 48
Flow rate, 104–105
    calculation, 140
Fluid balance, 34, 105–110, 106 (table)–109 (table)
Formula reference sheet, 139
Formulary, 19
Fraser guidelines, 62

Gastro-oesophageal reflux disease (GORD), 147
Gate control theory of pain, 121
Gender, 53, 132
General Medical Council (GMC), 10, 19
General Pharmaceutical Council (GPhC), 10
General sales list medicines (GSLs), 10, 11
Generic name, 45, 64
Genomics, 36, 129–130
Gillick competence, 62
Global action for Trans Equality (GATE), 132
Glyceryl trinitrate (GTN), 48, 70
Gut microbiome, 32, 126

Haemorrhoids, 32
Half-life, 33, 49–50
Health Act 2006, 2009, 14
Health and Safety Act 1974, 16–17
Health and Social Care Act 2008,
    17–18

Healthcare
    addressing inequality, 131
    antimicrobial resistance (AMR), 125–127
    Artificial intelligence (AI), 130
    challenges for, 125
    diagnostic systems, 129
    drug misuse, 127–128
    gender, 132
    genomics, 129–130
    health, global threats to, 128
    healthy lifestyle choices, 130
    healthy weight, 131
    immunisation, 127
    innovative medicine delivery, 129
    learning disability, 132–133
    mental health, 131
    new medicine development, 128–129
    opportunities for, 128
    political agenda, 128
    public perception, 127
    reducing alcohol consumption, 131
    refugees and migrants, 131
    smoking cessation, 130
    social prescribing, 131
Health, global threats to, 128
Healthy lifestyle choices, 130
Healthy weight, 131
HMG-CoA reductase inhibitors, 130
Homeostatic functions, 34
Homoeostasis, 27
    body systems, 30 (figure)
Human body
    chemical digestion, 32
    constituents, 25–28
    digestive system, 32
    first pass metabolism, 33
    immune system, 35
    inflammation, 35
    integrated body systems, 28–31
    liver, 33
    lymphocytes, 35
    mechanical digestion, 32
    pathogens, 35
    phagocytes, 35
    renal function, 34
Human Immunological Virus (HIV), 132
Human Medicines Regulations (HMSO) 2012, 15–16
Hypersensitive reactions, 75

Iatrogenic, 73
Immune system, 35
Immunisation, 76, 127
Immunological response, 8, 54, 72
Imperial weight conversion, 88
Implied consent, 61
Independent prescribers, 19
Inequality, 131
Inflammation, 33, 35, 51, 121
Inflammatory symptoms, 122
Informed consent, 61, 62
Infusion rates, 103, 107

Inhalation, 47, 53, 69, 71
Inhaler, 6, 71
Innovative medicine delivery, 129
International Digital Health and AI Research
    Collaborative (I-DAIR), 130
Interphase, 28
Interstitial space, 28
Intracellular, 27
Intramuscular, 15, 35, 68, 72, 97
Intravenous, 35, 64, 67, 68
Ion channels, 50, 52
Ions, 48, 52, 122

Labelling, 11, 73
    requirements, 11
Lasting power of attorney (LPA), 62
Laxatives, 122
Learning disability, 132–133
Legislation, 6, 8, 12, 18, 20
Liberty protection safeguards, 62
Lipid-soluble drugs, 34, 49
Liver, 33, 35, 48, 50, 51, 53, 74
Lymphocytes, 35

Malnutrition Universal Screening Tool (MUST), 95
    (figure)–146 (figure)
Margin of safety, 51
Massachusetts Institute of Technology (MIT), 129
Mathematical principles, 2, 84–85
Mechanical digestion, 32
Medical emergency, 35, 75
Medication management, modern age
    complementary and alternative medicines (CAMs),
        124–125
    healthcare. See Healthcare
    social prescribing, 125
    symptoms, 120–123
Medicine, 7–8, 10, 13, 20, 34, 44, 46–55, 64, 73, 128–129, 132
Medicine and Healthcare products Regulatory
    Agency (MHRA), 73, 129
Medicines Act 1968, 10–12, 11
Medicines management principles/practice
    calculating dose according to weight, 140
    calculating number of tablets required, 139
    calculating solutions/injections, 140
    calculating volume of fluid, 140
    case studies, 141–153
    converting units, 139
    drip rate calculation, 140
    flow rate calculation, 140
    formula reference sheet, 139
Mental health, 35, 37, 61, 74, 131
Metabolism, 2, 33, 35, 47, 49, 54, 75
Metric system, 85
Misuse of Drugs Act 1971, 12
Misuse of Drugs (designation) Order 2018
    Amendment, 13–14
Misuse of Drugs Regulations 2001, 12
Mitigate against, 9
Mitotic phase, 28
Morphine, 54, 66–67, 121
Multidisciplinary team, 7, 18–21, 68, 74

National Early Warning Scores, 126
National Institute of Health and Care Excellence
    (NICE), 13, 126, 129, 131
Nausea, 12, 122, 131, 134
Nearest whole number, 88–89
Near-misses, 17
Nebulisers, 71
Nervous system, 29, 74, 121
Neurogenic inflammation, 121
Never events, 17
New medicine development, 128–129
NHS Healthy Weight Calculator, 90
Nociceptive, 120
Non-medical prescribers, 19
Non-steroidal anti-inflammatory drugs (NSAIDs), 33,
    51, 121
Number fractions, 92–94
Nursing and Midwifery Council (NMC), 6
Nursing and Midwifery order 2001, 10
Nursing associates
    accountability, 9–10
    law and, 8–9
    responsibility, 9–10
Nutritional status, 54

Obesity, 54, 122, 131
Off-licence, 10
One-stop dispensing, 20
Onset of action, 45, 50, 52, 68
Opiates, 121–122
Opportunities, 2, 120, 128–131
Oral medication, 32, 68

Palliative care, 121, 128
Paracetamol, 7, 37, 45, 56, 98, 121–122
Parenteral, 11, 67, 95
Passive diffusion, 47, 48 (figure)
Pathogens, 35
Pathology/medical conditions, 54
Pathophysiology, 36
Patient group directions (PGDs), 19
Patient-specific direction, 19
Peak concentration, 50
Percentages, 94–96
Peristalsis, 32
Personal protective clothing (PPE), 72
Phagocytes, 35
Pharmacists, 20
Pharmacodynamics, 2, 45, 50–52
Pharmacogenomics, 53
Pharmacokinetics, 2, 36, 45, 47–50, 52,
    54, 65
Pharmacological principles
    administration, 44
    body does to medicine, 47–50
    medicinal effects, factors influencing, 53–55
    medicines uses, 46–47
    naming medicines, 45–46
    pharmacodynamics, 45, 50–52
    pharmacokinetics, 45, 47–50
    pharmacotherapeutics, 45
Pharmacotherapeutics, 45

Pharmacovigilance, 73, 129
Pharmacy medicines (P-medicines), 11
Pinocytosis, 48
Placebo effect, 54, 125
Placenta, 49, 75
Political agenda, 128
Polypharmacy, 34, 53, 125
Portal circulation, 48
Prescribing, 10, 12, 14, 19, 36, 53, 75, 125, 127, 131
Prescription-only medicines (POMs), 11
Prophylactic administration, 46
Proprietary name, 45–46, 64
Prostaglandins, 51, 121
Protons, 48
Pruritus, 122
Public Health England (PHE), 130, 136
Public perception, 127
Pyrexia, 122
Pyrogens, 122

Ratios, 96–98
Receptors, 28, 50, 122
Recognition, 35, 37, 75, 126, 131
Recommended International Nonproprietary
    Name (rINN), 46
Rectal, 32, 69, 72
Refugees and migrants, 131
Resuscitation Council (UK), 75
Rights
    allergy check, 65
    documentation, 65
    dose, 64
    effectiveness, 65
    medicine, 64
    medicines, 63
    patient, 64
    route, 65
    time, 64–65
Risk management, 17, 18
Royal Pharmaceutical Society (RPS), 82

Safe medicines administration
    adverse drug reactions (ADR), 73
    anaphylaxis, 75–77
    drug interaction, 74–75
    ethical considerations, 61–63
    patients' rights, 61–63
    procedures, 70–72
    rights of, 63–67
    routes of administration, 67–70
Safety critical medicines, 66
Schedules and classes, 12, 21
Secure stationery, 19
Sepsis, 126, 127, 133
Serious adverse events, 17
Signs, 7, 26, 37, 73, 105
Smoking cessation, 130
Social prescribing, 125, 131
Spacer, 69, 71
Specificity, 51
Subcutaneous, 35, 68–69, 72
Suffixes, 46
Supplementary prescribing, 19
Supply, 11, 19, 35, 47
Symptoms, 7, 11, 17, 32, 34, 37, 47, 51,
    64, 73, 123

Teratogenesis, 75
Thalamus, 121
Therapeutic administration, 47
Therapeutic index, 51
Tolerance, 54
Topically, 67
Tort law, 10
Transdermal, 35, 69
Transport systems, 28

UK Resuscitation Council algorithm, 2021, 75, 76
    (figure)
Units of measurement, 72, 82, 85–88
Unlicensed, 10, 13, 19
Urinary tract infection (UTI), 149
Urticaria, 123

Vaccine hesitancy, 2, 127
Vaginal routes, 68, 70
Vicarious liability, 2, 9, 21
Vomiting, 32, 54, 100, 122

Yellow card, 73–74, 77

Printed in the USA
CPSIA information can be obtained
at www.ICGtesting.com
CBHW080851180524
8518CB00018B/31

9 781529 623017